Margie L. Cristofaro
33711-141 Pl. S.E.
Auburn,WA 98002

NO-PILL
NO-RISK
BIRTH
CONTROL

NO-PILL NO-RISK BIRTH CONTROL

by
Nona Aguilar

Rawson, Wade Publishers, Inc. • New York

Library of Congress Cataloging in Publication Data

Aguilar, Nona.
    No-pill, no-risk birth control.

    Includes index.
        1. Rhythm method (Birth control). 2. Ovulation—Detection. 3. Cervix mucus. 4. Body temperature—Measurement.
5. Menstrual cycle. 6. Fertility, Human. I. Title.
RG136.5.A38   613.9′434   79-55463
ISBN 0-89256-118-1

Published simultaneously in Canada by McClelland
    and Stewart, Ltd.
Manufactured in the United States of America
Composition by American–Stratford Graphic Services,
    Brattleboro, Vermont
Printed and bound by Fairfield Graphics,
    Fairfield, Pennsylvania
Designed by Gene Siegel

Eighth Printing April 1984

This book is for T.H.F. and for the 400 men and women who allowed me to know so much about a deeply intimate part of their marital lives.

Acknowledgments

While I am listed author of this book, the Latin *et al.* belongs after my name. Many men and women contributed expertise and counsel, not only answering questions, but also reviewing and correcting many chapters while the manuscript was in progress.

Two are responsible for pointing me in the direction of the psychological and emotional effects of natural family planning: Maxine Lewis, health editor of *Family Circle* magazine, and Helen Paul, R.N., of Holy Name Hospital, Teaneck, New Jersey.

Two men made research information available to me: Paul Marx, O.S.B., Ph.D., director of the Human Life Center at St. John's University in Collegeville, Minnesota, and Lawrence Kane of the Human Life and Natural Family Planning Foundation in Washington, D.C. Mary Kay Williams, also of the Foundation, offered a great deal of direct assistance. In addition, her well-edited book (in collaboration with William A. Uricchio), *Proceedings of a Research Conference on Natural Family Planning,* was immensely helpful.

I depended heavily on the formulations and guidelines developed by Dr. Josef Roetzer of Voecklabruck,

Austria. Dr. Roetzer took time to write answering questions and was also available to me over several transatlantic telephone calls. Still, if there are any errors, they belong to me—with apologies to Dr. Roetzer.

Two who have developed important teaching materials on their own were consultants on this book. They are Carman and Jean Fallace, directors of Family Life Promotion of New York, Inc., and authors of *The Joy in Planning Your Family* (private printing).

John F. Kippley has contributed valuable help and always gave thoughtful, serious advice when I needed it. He is the author of several excellent books on family planning, including *The Art of Natural Family Planning*, which was co-authored with his wife, Sheila Kippley. John Kippley is also director of the Couple to Couple League (Cincinnati, Ohio), the largest and most effective natural family planning teaching organization in the United States.

Two doctors' valuable insights inform many portions of this book: Herbert Ratner, M.D., editor of *Child and Family* (see Appendix C for subscription information), and Teaneck, New Jersey, gynecologist James Fox, M.D.

Psychiatrist George M. Maloof (San Francisco) spent many hours working over material in the manuscript that, alas, had to be excised because of the total length of the book. I'm sure that the deletion pained me more than it pained Dr. Maloof.

Two doctors answered my questions throughout the year that I worked on the manuscript, and reviewed many of the chapters, offering suggestions and criticisms: Lester B. Anderman, M.D. (Los Angeles), and Edward F. Keefe, M.D. (New York). Indeed, sound suggestions from Dr. Anderman prompted several substantive manuscript revisions.

Virginia D. Gager, editor of the *International Review of Natural Family Planning*, made meticulous corrections and thoughtful suggestions on the chapters explaining the methods. Mrs. Gager is considered by many authorities to be the best editor in the field of modern, scientific NFP and I've relied on many of her recommendations in writing chapters 3, 4, and 5. Also, the chapter on infertility was written on Mrs. Gager's recommendation.

Bonnie Manion, R.N., of the Human Life Center at St. John's University in Collegeville, Minnesota, is a superb teacher. She not only made extensive corrections on the manuscript, she also stayed "on call," answering all my questions during the months of writing.

Charles G. Mills, Farley Clinton, Marian J. Amft, and David Wilkinson, Ph.D., made valuable suggestions. Charles Mills, in particular, worked intensively on sections of the manuscript, helping to shape material that, in the end, had to be cut because of the length of the original manuscript. The suggestions from these four were always provoking; only a few were ignored.

Dr. Robert M. Nakamura of the University of Southern California Medical Center (Los Angeles) made a number of pertinent recommendations and showed enormous patience in answering a stream of questions.

I am deeply grateful to Gloria Roberts of the Katherine Dexter McCormick Library of the Planned Parenthood—World Population Information & Education Department. All the information in this book concerning the problems and side effects of contraception and sterilization came from the well-kept files of this library. Mrs. Roberts was always extremely helpful in pointing me in the right direction to find precisely the statistic I required.

Two people substantially lifted the burden of writing: Patrick W. Garrard lent me an office complete with a photocopying machine, and Edward T. Bomar helped get this book finished and *out* to the publisher.

Some 250 men and women—all users of natural family planning—shared their experiences with me in private, personal interviews. Another 157 returned detailed, six-page essay-type questionnaires telling me about their experiences in this intimate area of their marriage. It is to these people that I owe my deepest thanks for my awareness that natural family planning is a life style that happens to include highly effective birth control.

Contents

xvi   *Contents*

Foreword

This book describes an effective birth control method that requires no drugs, chemicals, or barrier devices. There is only one requirement for its use: understanding.

Although the subject of reproduction has been studied for centuries, information on the cyclic levels of the reproductive hormones in serum during the menstrual cycle was first published only ten years ago. Since then, research concerning the pituitary, ovary, and their end-organs has been published at a fantastic rate. Possibly greater than ninety percent of the total volume of information on reproduction has been published in just this last decade. This information boom is becoming difficult for even the experts to handle.

That's why one of the things that most impresses me about this book is the author's ability to make biological and scientific facts clear and understandable. The extensive description of the many methods that measure the variables during the reproductive cycle is necessary and well done. The discussion and use of anecdotes to explain the results of these methods are easy to follow and understand. The section on nursing, which was a lost art for a time, is very informative for new parents. Indeed, as I read this book I kept wondering why we in academia, and the scientific community at large, can't seem to be able to impart information on reproduction as clearly and as concisely as the author does.

But besides the clarity of her presentation, Nona Aguilar has done an excellent job of asking the relevant questions. I am often amazed that many in the so-called sophisticated world of academic research are content merely with answers. They refuse to recognize that we desperately need good questions as well; such questions are the foundation of a better understanding of reproduction. In this regard, *No-Pill, No-Risk Birth Control* is a good lesson to all. Miss Aguilar is able to show readers the whole forest, and at the same time knows how to examine various trees calmly. This is obviously in contradistinction to some who hurry to examine the veins in a leaf but have limited interest in the nature of the tree, and no interest whatsoever in the forest.

Throughout this foreword I have constantly focused my attention on reproduction. The reason is obvious: the relevant information is applicable to both the fertile and the infertile couple. But I can't stress the word "couple" enough. When both the man and the woman learn about the physiology of the reproductive system, there is an important basis for better understanding between them. It is this larger area of understanding that Nona Aguilar addresses particularly well.

Before concluding, I want to point out that my reading in the area of human reproduction is almost exclusively limited to medical journals, monographs, and reports on ongoing research. But I can say that I feel fortunate that a set of strange and wonderful circumstances brought this book my way.

Robert M. Nakamura
University of Southern California
Medical Center
Los Angeles, California

I

Male and Female Fertility: A Shared Adventure

I

The Story Behind This Book

The book you are holding will open your eyes to a completely different kind of birth control: totally natural methods.

Natural methods are highly effective—as effective as the Pill. Yet no drugs, devices, or surgery is ever required. The methods depend entirely on nature.

Is this dependence uncertain? Unreliable?

No, it isn't.

It has always been known that every act of intercourse does not result in pregnancy. A woman is periodically fertile, infertile, and then fertile once again. This is a natural rhythm, a natural cycle experienced throughout a woman's reproductive decades.

In its truest form, it is the rhythm of the life-bearing force of the human race. It has the power to dictate whether or not a child will come into existence.

Certainly you yourself know the power of this force: it once resulted in your conception; it can result in the conception of your children.

But is it possible that your body could be so receptive to human life one day, not at all on another day, and yet give no sign whatsoever of this profound alteration?

As you will learn from reading this book, it is neither possible nor the case.

A woman's body signals very clearly whether or not conception is possible on any particular day. And the reason natural birth control is so effective is that it depends on natural fertility indicators. To utilize natural methods effectively you must simply learn to read these indicators.

If you wish to conceive, engage in intercourse when your body becomes fertile and receptive to life. If you wish to postpone or avoid conception, the fertility indicators will tell you when to abstain.

Your body won't lie or mislead you. That's why these methods are as reliable as the Pill or the most effective of the sterilization procedures.

However, natural methods do have one important requirement for effective use: *at their core, all natural methods are cooperative ventures.*

With these methods, birth control is no longer "the man's job" or "the woman's job." *Both* use the methods—or neither uses them.

The importance of cooperation in natural birth control is indicated by the language used to describe the method. *"We* use natural family planning" is the only phrase that can describe this new situation adequately. It takes a plural pronoun. In contrast, pronouns used to describe artificial birth control are always singular. *"He* uses a condom," *"I* take the Pill," are common examples.

At first glance, cooperation appears to be a sham. Rather, it seems that in this important area of sex, nature is refusing to cooperate with *us.* After all, couples who rely on natural methods must cope with the times when they aren't able to have sexual intercourse. And while this is true, there is something curious that happens to a couple in the process of cooperating with nature: in the end, the two can become more fully spouses, friends, partners—they can become most fully *lovers*.

I didn't always believe this. My first awareness of it came suddenly. I was given the name of a nurse connected with a New Jersey hospital who had taught natural methods for ten years in the Philippines and had been involved with a New Jersey program for about three years. I called for an interview.

When I arrived at the appointed time for the interview, research notebook in hand, I was surprised to find that additional guests had volunteered to come: seven men and women were waiting, including a physician.

These men and women were all using natural methods. Four had used artificial methods in the past. All had come to meet me, to tell me their stories.

As they told me how they had learned about natural methods and the deep effects these methods had had on their love relationships, I became aware that the *psychological dimensions of artificial birth control methods and natural methods were totally different.*

As these seven men and women spoke, the words I'd read in the psychological literature concerning birth control ceased to be cant and jargon and became flesh and blood, emotions and feelings.

For the first time I began to understand what was meant when I read that natural methods fostered couple communication, that artificial methods were at least a hindrance to this vital exchange, and more often a complete block.

All at once I knew—*really* knew—what was meant by many women's complaints that they had been turned into sex objects by men. With incredible clarity, I saw that natural family planning could restore both personhood and equality to women.

In sudden, bold relief, I recognized one of the inner springs of sexual boredom and ennui—the special complaint of so many men and women.

I had heard words and phrases like "growing closer," "becoming more intimate," "falling more in love," spoken by many professionals involved with natural family planning. Though the words sounded theoretical, I had dutifully written them into my research notebook.

For the first time the words were written into my heart.

That interview completely changed my life.

In saying that, I don't refer to the two years I spent interviewing hundreds of men and women from coast to coast about their experiences after switching from contraception to natural family planning. The change I refer to is one that involves a radical revolution of my thinking about male/female relations, sex—*good* sex, the dynamics of love, and the makings of a really lasting relationship.

So while this book is primarily about fertility control by natural family planning (NFP), it is also about the astonishing array of beneficent consequences and rewards that are yours when you and your mate surrender to a natural love style and life style.

2

The Reason We Hate Contraceptives

Why do natural methods seem to make such a difference? The very first person I ever spoke to about the subject indicated the reason.

And curiously, that person was a man.

Since birth control has been considerably more than less a woman's job, it has been a consistent surprise to me that some of the best insights concerning natural methods vis-à-vis artificial ones come from men. As it turned out, that man's perceptive observation about contraception has been confirmed to me in interview after interview with couples around the country as well as through extensive reading of the medical literature. In addition, I've analyzed 157 detailed essay-type confidential questionnaires from couples relying on natural family planning, most of whom had used contraception in the past.

And this earthshaking observation was—and is—fairly obvious: *every contraceptive involves a "shock" of some kind to either the woman or the man, or to both. But usually, depending on the artificial method used, one partner has to absorb most, or even all, of the shock.*

Of course, the shock this man referred to wasn't an electrical bolt, a physical blow, or an emotional trauma.

7

Rather, the shock he meant involves an interruption of natural processes—but an interruption that includes a measure of disturbance, physiologically or psychologically, and sometimes both.

The Condom

The condom is the only known barrier method that demands attention by both partners. If the man has an erection, genital-genital contact must be avoided. There may be live sperm in the pre-coital fluid that could survive in favorable external vaginal mucus, ultimately swimming "upstream" to the site of conception, the Fallopian tubes. Thus, both the man and the woman must be alert for the appropriate interval during love-making to apply the contraceptive.

When the most propitious time arrives, it is best to try to make the placing of the condom part of the love play; otherwise, it is interruptive. Indeed, no matter how playfully a couple tries to make the condom a third partner in love-making, most complain that it's still an interruption.

Other matters require attention. For example, unless the man is using a nipple-type, the condom must be drawn over the erect penis so that about a half-inch of the tip remains empty to receive the ejaculate.

Does relaxation of vigilance begin after orgasm? Alas, not even then. Continuing attention is demanded, since the contraceptive must be held right at the base of the still erect penis as the man withdraws so that no semen accidentally spills on the woman's genitals.

All these matters are really disturbances of what could otherwise be a splendid, unencumbered, exuberant sexual exchange between a man and a woman. It is in this sense that the condom involves a shock to both partners, since there is an interruption of natural processes involving physiological—and even psychological—disturbances during the act of intercourse.

But what is worse, the above "shock" listing doesn't even include what is potentially the biggest shock to condom users: unexpected pregnancy.

Reliability. Some effectiveness figures suggest that of 100 couples relying on condoms alone for a year, only 3 would conceive. Other studies suggest that as many as 30 couples would conceive.

Biostatistics are tricky for an obvious reason: the human element. And nowhere is it more capricious than in the area of sex and contraception.

Motivation is essential to the effectiveness of any contraceptive method. It is also the reason why contraception statistics exist in at least two different forms: theoretical effectiveness and extended-use effectiveness.

The theoretical effectiveness of a method refers to its maximum effectiveness when used properly, following the instructions for its use at *every single intercourse.* Used properly at every intercourse, the condom is at least 97 percent effective. But extended-use effectiveness figures take into account *all* users—those who use the method perfectly *as well as* the careless users, including those who fail to use the contraceptive. So the astonishingly high figure of thirty conceptions is a use-effectiveness figure. The careless couples, the couples with little or no motivation to use the condom properly—or at all—are included.

Other Barrier Methods

For all of the reasons mentioned, it is not surprising that the condom is not a favorite among couples who rely on barrier methods for artificial birth control. Instead, more couples opt for either the diaphragm or foam.

To be sure, the diaphragm has *its* drawbacks. It must be "fitted" by a doctor or nurse practitioner, inserted less than two hours before intercourse with appropriate spermicidal cream or jelly, and additional spermicide must be applied before every subsequent intercourse. The contraceptive must be left in place for at least six to eight hours after intercourse; upon removal, it must be washed, dusted with cornstarch or talc, and stored for the next use. So although it requires less attention *during* love-making than the condom, the diaphragm also affects spontaneity.

There is another matter: use of the diaphragm devolves solely on the woman, and contraception is no longer a joint venture between a man and a woman (as the condom can be).

In recognizing that the woman carries this burden, it is often suggested that the husband help his wife insert the device as part of the preliminary love play to enhance the couple's sense of sharing and intimacy. This seems to be one of those nice-in-theory-BUT suggestions. A wife summarizes the experience in one terse sentence: "It turned us both off."

In contrast, spermicidal foam can involve mutual effort. The product comes in a can and combines a spermicide with an inert chemical base that acts as a medium to hold the chemical spermicide in place against the cervix. It's important to shake the can vigorously to insure that a good "bubble barrier" is formed, one that is thoroughly mixed with spermicide. Thus, the man can shake the can, fill the applicator, and apply the product inside the woman's vagina.

Shock factors are relatively minor. One complaint is that effective use of foam demands insertion about a half-hour before coitus, since the spermicide begins to lose effectiveness after approximately thirty minutes. This requirement may affect spontaneity, but at least it doesn't interrupt the actual act of intercourse.

Some men and women also complain that the foam

causes a burning sensation. Also, there are reports of penile and vaginal irritation attributable to the foams, although frequently a simple switch to a different brand takes care of the problem.

Couples who enjoy oral stimulation complain about the unpleasant taste of foams. Their use may limit oral forms of stimulation and pleasure—an unwelcome "intrusion" to some couples.

Effectiveness. While foam *seems* to be slightly less effective than the diaphragm, most authorities give both methods a theoretical effectiveness rating of 97 percent. A possible reason why foam is "considered" less effective is that its various *use*-effectiveness figures reflect as many as a third more unplanned pregnancies than the diaphragm: 30 pregnancies per 100 woman users versus 20 to 25 for the diaphragm. Researchers are really not sure why the extended-use-effectiveness figures show such a wide spread.

Doubling Technique

There is an obvious technique for dramatically increasing the reliability of barrier contraceptive methods: doubling. A frequent "double" is the condom and foam. Another is the diaphragm combined with either foam or the condom.

While contraceptive reliability is radically increased by doubling, the "shock" factors may also rise. However, they don't *necessarily* rise, since one method can offset the disadvantages of the other. The condom-foam combination is a perfect example of this.

First, foam must be applied just prior to love-making, affecting spontaneity. But then genital-genital contact is not a serious matter if the foam is in place. True, actual love-making must be interrupted so that the condom can be placed, but if the man finds foam irritating, he is protected by the prophylactic.

So for all its drawbacks—and some of its advantages— "doubling" draws a number of highly motivated couples. But couples using this method must be disciplined and very motivated.

Total Body Shock: The Pill

When the Pill made its debut approximately twenty years ago, only the palm branches were missing; the hosannas and cheers were certainly there. At last, a method that had everything!

No more leaping out of bed to get "trussed up" with a diaphragm!

No more opening the night table drawer—*always* when things were just getting good—to grope for a condom!

The hormones could be swallowed morning or evening or at some other regularly scheduled time apart from, and independent of, intercourse. The sex act itself was completely free of interruption; the shock factor was (apparently) nonexistent. Even more appealing, the theoretical effectiveness of the original Pill approached 100 percent. The Pill takers lined up—by the tens of millions.

So why, despite all this apparent satisfaction, has there been a sudden drop in the number of Pill takers?

There is a simple answer to this. According to Teaneck, New Jersey, gynecologist James Fox, we have passed the fifteen-year latency period on the Pill. Early suspicions have become confirmed fact. As a result, more is being said against the Pill, *not* because anyone is picking at the drug, but rather, because there is demonstrably more to pick *at*.

Metabolic changes. It has been known since the late sixties that the Pill affects the metabolic functions in a woman's body. Approximately fifty metabolic changes occur in the bodies of women who swallow the Pill daily. With such profound alterations attributable to the Pill, it is not surprising that it seems to be:

- carcinogenic;
- a (sometimes fatal) blood-clotting factor;
- a factor that doubles a woman's chance of developing gall bladder diseases if used continuously for only two years;
- a causative agent in increased heart and limb defects in a child whose mother unwittingly becomes pregnant and continues taking the drug.

Other "minor" side effects include nausea, weight changes, and ankle swelling. Migraine, epilepsy, and kidney or heart disease symptoms may worsen. Your hair may stop growing, fall out, or grow more abundantly and luxuriously.

The point is, the Pill *does* affect you. The Pill shock is enormous, and we are just beginning to recognize its enormity.

The results of a long-term study that began in 1968 and ultimately involved some 46,000 women of childbearing age in the United Kingdom were reported in the October 8, 1977, issue of *The Lancet,* a distinguished British medical journal read throughout the world. The study concentrated on deaths—*only* deaths—and their causes.

In contrast, studies that have attempted to link the Pill with disease conditions have run into an "overreporting" problem. Were, for example, migraines, dizziness, aching legs, depression, loss of sex drive, nausea, sore breasts, and other problems *really* caused by taking the Pill, or were these complaints psychological in origin? Even in the British study in question, examiners did not pin the deaths on the Pill. They merely recorded death statistics—numbers of deaths and their causes. Two inescapable facts stood out prominently:

- The total death rate for women who had ever used the Pill at any time in their lives was increased by 40 percent.
- The increased death rate was due to a surprisingly wide range of vascular diseases—conditions that were considerably more varied than had ever been suspected.

This last fact is considered to be very telling. Women who took the oral contraceptives received medical "clearance" for existent or pre-existent heart and vascular disease conditions. They were *not* part of the most-are-healthy-some-aren't general population.

The controls were.

But despite the fact that Pill takers were healthier than the general population, their death rates were conspicuously higher.

Even more disturbing, according to the study, "The present findings suggest that the risk of circulatory diseases increases with the duration of oral-contraceptive use and *may persist after the pill is discontinued.*" (Emphasis added.)

Certainly this is a different view than the "rubberband" theory that has prevailed—the notion that mere discontinuation of the Pill is enough for the woman's body to snap back to its pre-Pill condition.

There was one surprise finding. Although the controls became pregnant more often than the Pill takers, the study found that ". . . the increased mortality associated with oral contraceptive use is much greater than the excess mortality . . . associated with the larger number of pregnancies in the controls."*

In other words, Pill taking to prevent pregnancy is riskier than pregnancy.

Taking chances. Despite these disturbing findings, many women continue to believe the it-won't-happen-to-me theory. Yet 1 in 5,000 who have ever taken the Pill will die every year from circulatory diseases. Long-time Pill critic Dr. Herbert Ratner, a public health physician and medical editor in Oak Park, Illinois, says this death rate is one of "epidemic proportions."

Some women feel that they can protect themselves—in effect, reduce their risk—by frequent examination and checking. There is one problem with this approach: examination will detect Pill problems *after* they've occurred, but not before.

So we come back to the point made at the opening of this chapter: Every contraceptive involves a shock of some kind. The Pill shock is pharmacological and physiological. Its impact on the delicate body mechanism can be so profound that it is not unfair to suggest that the Pill shock *can be lethal for some women.*

The "Localized" Shock: The IUD

Many women have by-passed the total body shock of the Pill and accepted the more "localized" shock of the intrauterine device (IUD) . Most models apparently affect only the uterus, although a few, such as the copper-bearing

---

* An epidemiological study by Valerie Beral published two years later in the September 15, 1979, *British Medical Journal* drew the same conclusions, noting that in 1975 ". . . it is estimated that there were more deaths at ages 25–44 years in England and Wales from adverse effects of oral contraceptive use than from all complications of pregnancy, delivery, and the puerperium combined."

and progesterone-loaded IUDs, may have systemic effects that is, effects throughout the body. *In actual fact, all IUDs have potentially systemic effects.*

Dangers. Occasionally a perforation of the uterus occurs at insertion. However, perforations can occur any-time—days, weeks, months, or even years—after the initial insertion. But since the uterus was not designed to be occupied by foreign objects, there are not enough nerve fibers in the uterus to alert the IUD wearer to potential problems through the pain mechanism. A woman's body can enter a state of medical emergency, its owner serenely unaware of the fact.

Other difficulties. Overall, nearly 70 percent of all IUD users have had their devices removed before the fourth "insertion anniversary." But what is really striking is that nearly half of the women in that 70 percent group requested IUD removal *within one year of the insertion.*

Why so soon? What are the problems? Here's one woman's experience:

> When I got my IUD I thought yippee! No more Pills, no more migraines, no more aching legs. My only "job" was to check the string regularly to make sure that I hadn't accidentally lost my IUD.
>
> But the first thing I noticed was very bad cramps during my period. I had never had any before. Also, I noticed that the flow was much heavier.
>
> The next problem developed gradually. Before I got my IUD my periods lasted about four or five days. Right after I got it, they began to last seven, eight, or nine days. Then month by month they lasted even longer. By the time I had the IUD removed, I was bleeding almost constantly. I had worn it less than fourteen months.

The woman's excessive bleeding and cramping are some of the more common IUD problems acknowledged by doctors. Others include:

- Imbedding of the IUD in the uterine wall—a problem that may require surgical attention.
- Perforation of the uterus—a surgical emergency.
- Anemia and other illnesses caused by blood losses associated with heavy menstrual bleeding provoked by the IUD.
- Pelvic inflammations and infections.

The last complaint is believed to occur because the IUD string may act as a wick, drawing harmful bacteria into the uterus. Indeed, some infection problems have been so serious that women have undergone major surgery to remove a part (an ovary, a tube) or even all of their reproductive organs. *Contraceptive Technology* co-author, Robert A. Hatcher, M.D., reports that some clinicians consider "desire for a future pregnancy if a woman has never been pregnant" as a contraindication for insertion of the device.

According to a report by Morton Mintz of *The Washington Post,* IUD-related problems are so prevalent that army obstetrician-gynecologist Major Russell J. Thomsen scored one drug company for promoting a device by using a "pathetic" study involving only 606 women in which the admitted complication rate was 25 percent *even though* one-fifth of all the women were lost to follow-up.

IUD action. Exactly *how* the IUD works as a contraceptive is not known with absolute certainty. In a 1972 paper prepared under the supervision of members of the faculty of the Mayo Graduate School of Medicine (University of Minnesota), Thomas W. Hilgers, M.D., notes the following:

There is no evidence that the IUD consistently prevents fertilization. On the other hand, it seems likely that fertilization occurs with normal or near normal frequency in the presence of the IUD. . . . On the basis of direct uterine observation with the glass fiber hysteroscope in 55 patients wearing IUD's, Sakurabayashi *et al.* concluded that the "fertilized ovum" was rapidly expelled from the uterine cavity.

If Dr. Hilgers is correct, many incompletely understood elements fall into place.

One matter that has been noted—and been a matter of concern—is the high number of pregnancies that occurred even when the IUD was in place. This may mean that pregnancies occur regularly when the IUD is in place, but that the conceptus is expelled because of the disturbing effects of the IUD on the uterine lining.

In other words, the action of the IUD is almost certainly abortifacient.

Sometimes the conceptus resists immediate expulsion and does manage to implant itself. Still, it usually can't develop normally with the IUD trying to occupy the same space, and a miscarriage is likely. IUD miscarriages are significantly more dangerous to the mother than normal ones because infection risks are substantially greater. A number of maternal deaths have been caused by such infections, according to Dr. Hilgers.

There are also several-times-normal rates of ectopic (tubular) pregnancies and septic abortions (caused by infection) reported among IUD users—all life-threatening medical emergencies. IUD-associated deaths have also been reported.

It is in this sense that any IUD must be considered to have potentially systemic effects on the total organism.

The IUD shock to the body is sometimes as great—though of a different nature—as the Pill shock.

The Surgical Shock: Female Sterilization

Charts listing various birth control options usually suggest that sterilization may have "minor complications." This hardly tells the whole story, since deaths have been reported and there is even a *death rate figure* for various procedures.

"Band-Aid" surgery. One sterilization procedure that has received a lot of publicity recently is the so-called "Band-Aid" procedure, hailed as an "easy" surgical method. Any surgical procedure has risks (pneumonia, major blood pressure drop precipitating heart attack or stroke, cardiac arrest, etc.) and the "Band-Aid" has these risks plus special ones of its own.

Gas is introduced into the abdomen, blowing it up like a balloon to separate the bowel from the abdominal wall. The surgeon then makes a small incision to permit insertion of the laparoscope—a tube with a lens on one end and a light on the other. Peering through the lens, he can pick up the Fallopian tubes with forceps and burn them with an electrical current. He withdraws the instrument, takes a small suture, and applies the famous Band-Aid.

The special problems? Inserting the needle into the abdomen sometimes punctures the bowel and causes peritonitis and abscess formation—a life-threatening situation.

After making the incision, the surgeon has only a limited field of vision: it is not unknown for a surgeon to damage the wrong structures accidentally or tear major blood vessels "poking around" for the Fallopian tubes. Also, the bowels have sometimes been burned (accidentally), causing acute peritonitis.

A November 23, 1973, New Republic Feature Syndicate release reported these cases involving the surgery:

- A woman died during the night from unrecognized bleeding. She was in her thirties.
- Another woman suffered a heart attack immediately after her abdomen was filled with gas.
- A woman was readmitted to a major hospital forty-eight hours after the surgery with acute peritonitis.

Doctors aren't always enthusiastic about the procedure either. Here's a portion of a letter on the subject written by Dr. H. P. Dunn, a leading New Zealand gynecologist with an international reputation:

I am fed up with these sterilization operations. We had three disasters, or major troubles, following the procedures this week.

The first young patient had her tubes tied at her fourth Caesarean (even though the uterine scar was sound) by a very competent young surgeon. Twelve hours later he called me to help him; she was bleeding into the abdominal cavity from a large spurting artery in the left tubal area and needed seven pints of blood. Twelve hours later she had a second collapse and had to be opened again—she was bleeding from the right tube operation! So I said to the residents: "Don't ever give patients the impression that this is a minor operation."

The next woman had had her tubes tied, then later wanted them re-opened—a difficult operation, but successful in this case. But she had a serious complication (ectopic pregnancy) and needed a third operation.

The third case was the usual excessive heavy

bleeding that dated exactly from the tubal ligation; at the age of only 34 she needed a hysterectomy.[1]

Dr. Dunn's dismay concerning sterilization arises from clinical experiences; Dr. Jacques-E. Rioux's dismay is a response to statistics. Writing in *The Journal of Reproductive Medicine* in December, 1977, Dr. Rioux called for a modern prospective study ". . . to find the real answers as to the long-term effects of female sterilizations." Dr. Rioux noted that the trend toward these procedures is growing. "Unfortunately," Dr. Rioux reported, "the medical profession cannot 'sell' sterilization as exempt from complications. . . . A review of the literature from 1951 to 1975 reveals an astounding range of cited incidence of acute morbidity (1.8% to 50%) and similar variations for long-range complications (2.5% to 52%)."

Statistics. In the August, 1975, issue of *The Journal of Reproductive Medicine* an article appeared entitled "Survey of Gynecologic Laparoscopy." The following is the last paragraph from that article: "The death rate reported in 1973–1974 (8/100,000) approaches the death rate attributed to the use of the birth control pill (3/100,000), the intrauterine device (4–5/100,000) and abortion (3–5/100,000). Additional refinements in technique will probably insure a narrowing of this gap."

A June, 1974, Hastings Center Report entitled "Voluntary Female Sterilization: Abuses, Risks and Guidelines" by Robert E. McGarrah, Jr., made several comparisons among hysterectomy, tubal ligation, and the Pill. At the time that the report was published, McGarrah noted that there were 31 Pill-related deaths per million women. In comparison, tubal ligation accounted for 1,000 deaths per million women and so did hysterectomy.

But the serious-complications rates were dramatically higher than the death rates. The Pill accounted for

600 serious complications per million women taking their daily swallows. But the tubal ligation rate was 15,000 per million women, and the serious complications from hysterectomy were ten times greater still: 150,000 per million women!

A more recent chart appeared in *Contraceptive Technology,* 1976–1977, on page 99. Here's a quick rundown on some of the mortality figures per 100,000 women (versus the million base figure used in the Hastings Center report) per year. (Note: no time frame was used in the Hastings report.)

> Oral contraceptives .. 0.3–3
> IUD 1.5
> Hysterectomy 300–500
> Laparoscopic tubal
>   ligation 12–50
> Abdominal 25
> Vaginal 150

(Note: Abdominal procedures include laparotomy, minilaparotomy, and laparoscopy. Vaginal procedures include colpotomy and culdoscopy.)

Other hazards. Although the chances of not surviving a sterilization procedure are small, the possibility does exist and would-be users of the procedures should be aware of this fact. They should also be aware that they are likely to have problems with *any* sterilization procedure selected.

Item: "A total of 374 patients were followed up for at least 10 years after tubal ligation, and 43% required further gynaecological treatment. Major gynaecological surgery was needed by 25%."[2]

Item: "The frequency of late sequelae in 454 patients sterilized by laparoscopy and diathermy or by abdominal tubal ligation was compared with that in 154 controls whose husbands had had a vasectomy. Results showed an increase in menstrual loss and pain with menstruation in the sterilized groups, especially if this had been done by diathermy and division under laparoscopic control. . . . 10 women subsequently required hysterectomy in the operative groups and 1 in the control group."[3]

Item: One month later the authors of the above study wrote an update in a November 15, 1975, letter published in *The Lancet.* Several points were made, including the following: "Since the study terminated one year ago, we are now aware of 20 women who have come to hysterectomy . . . and 1 in the control group."

Item: "Williams, Jones, and Merrill in their series of 200 patients at Vanderbilt University Hospital [found that] twenty-four per cent of their patients developed clinically significant gynecologic disorders following tubal ligation. The authors estimated that 31 per cent of the women undergoing tubal ligation would develop some significant gynecologic problem if followed for 10 years."[4]

Shock factor. Why do so many complications occur? Researchers are still not sure. There is a possibility that the ovarian blood supply is seriously disturbed in some unknown way when the tubes are cut, clipped, or cauterized. Also, it may be possible that certain hormonal functions—also unknown—are disrupted.

At any rate, it *is* known that about a quarter to a third of all women undergoing sterilization procedures will have some kind of problem, some of them serious enough to require hysterectomy. The minor complications—minor, of course, as long as *you* aren't the person suffering them—usually fall into one or two of the following categories reminiscent of the complications from the IUD:

- Heavy menstrual bleeding. Often the menstrual days increase and the flow becomes heavier. Some women develop anemia because of the loss of so much blood.
- Extreme discomfort and painful cramping during menstruation.
- Increased incidence of pelvic disease.

There is one ironic "minor" complication that some women suffer as a result of sterilization: painful, uncomfortable intercourse.

So the "shock" factors associated with a sterilization procedure are very high. Mortality rates for some of the procedures are 2, 3, 25, 150, even 300 times higher than mortality rates for either the Pill or the IUD!

Effectiveness. Despite all these risks, post-sterilization pregnancy rates are about 1 to 2 percent for most of the procedures, 5 percent with others. So while the procedure is theoretically 100 percent effective, in fact, the use-effectiveness rates are as low as 95 percent, since tubal reconnection may occur after surgery.

Although full-term pregnancies occur, ectopic pregnancies are more frequent, since the conceptus is sometimes "caught" in the tube when it only partially reconnects. Ectopic pregnancies can occur anytime after the procedure—months later, years later. But *because* she has been sterilized, the woman rarely suspects that she could possibly be pregnant: the rupture risk becomes even more serious—and dangerous.

That's why, all things considered, the sterilization "shock" is profound, even fatal.

The Incompletely Explored Shock: Vasectomy

It was all very puzzling.

The men were young, only in their twenties and thirties. They had all enjoyed apparent good health. Had they ever had surgery? The answer they gave was usually no.

Yet the men all displayed a puzzling array of medical problems, all of rather recent origin. They included thrombophlebitis, persistent fevers, enlargement of the lymph nodes, skin eruptions, and constantly recurring infections.

More serious problems included the development of hypoglycemia, blood clotting, and severe narcolepsy—a strange disorder in which the subject not only suddenly falls asleep at the most inappropriate times, but also has "spells" in which he loses all muscular control. Other symptoms that developed were even more incapacitating: acute multiple sclerosis and arthritis were two.

Dr. H. J. Roberts reported these cases in the *British Medical Journal*. In the same article, Dr. Roberts explained that as each young man came to consult him, he grew more and more perplexed by the symptoms and explored even further. "By questioning *every* individual [emphasis is Roberts's] with such unexplained features, a history of vasectomy prior to their onset has been uncovered when it was completely forgotten during routine query about previous surgery."[5]

"Completely forgotten." Those two words summarize the ease and simplicity of the vasectomy procedure: when asked about previous surgery, men who have been vasectomized barely remember it—or think to mention it.

The procedure. Certainly many doctors who are aware of the problems associated with female sterilization operations favor the idea of male sterilization by vasectomy.

And why not?

The procedure is considered to be relatively simple. It's a matter of tying (cutting or cauterizing) each vas near the testicles. The sperm cells are then prevented from mixing with the fluids produced by the seminal vesicles, prostate, and other glands. Most researchers indicate that after vasectomy there is no change in the quality or strength of subsequent orgasms.

Complication rates? Reportedly very low. In one study made at Houston's Baylor College of Medicine involving 2,711 vasectomies during the nineteen-month period between June 1, 1970, and January 1, 1972, the "major complications" rate was 4.1 percent and included adhesion problems, epididymitis, abscess formation, and hematomas.

In a study of 1,000 vasectomy operations performed at the Margaret Pyke Centre in London, 122 (or 12.2 percent) early post-operative complications were noted at the end of the first month, according to the study results published in the October 27, 1973, issue of the *British Medical Journal*. But overall, researchers were satisfied with results.

However, the procedures involved in working up the studies just mentioned *are not designed to reveal some of the possible systemic complications involved.* In fact, some of the possible problems (running fevers, lymph node enlargement, recurrent infection, etc.) are not generally associated with the sterilization at all. This evidence is considered to be merely associative, although according to a November 3, 1972, article in *Medical World News* entitled "Vasectomy complications aplenty," some urologists are beginning to take Dr. Roberts's report seriously. The reason? Urologists recognize the fact that it is really not known what happens to the spermatozoa that continue to be produced in the testes.

Effectiveness. There is agreement among professionals on two counts:

1. Some reversal operations have been successful, but most have not. Thus, the subject should always

assume that the procedure will be permanent.
2. Sometimes the procedure reverses itself!

In about 1 percent to 2 percent of the cases, the tubes reconnect ("spontaneous recanalization") and the man can impregnate once again.

In one case, recanalization occurred despite what could be considered triple fail-safe procedures: not only had a section of the vas been removed, but there had been a diathermic procedure with electrical current *plus* a doubling back of the ends before ligation with nonabsorbable sutures.

In another case, a man went through not one but *two* vasectomies . . . and continued to show a positive sperm count. The researchers reported wryly: "This man is now using condoms and is, understandably enough, disillusioned about the vasectomy procedure."[6]

But overall, the procedure is successful in about 98 or 99 percent of the cases. Moreover, men generally continue to report satisfaction with the sterilization when surveyed a year or so after the operation. For these reasons, among others, the couple who does not wish to have children is sometimes urged to choose male sterilization. At least there have been no reports of death.

The Contraceptive Future

After surveying modern methods, it becomes apparent that the higher the *use* effectiveness of an artificial method or surgical procedure, the greater the shock. Vasectomy may prove an exception to this generalization if Dr. Roberts's reports are eventually shown to be unfounded. On the other hand, the shock factors involved in modern methods of female contraception—the Pill and the IUD in particular—have become so great that epidemiologist

Valerie Beral has called for a new measurement category of female deaths. "Reproductive mortality," the proposed category, would include not only deaths from pregnancy-related complications, but also deaths from the adverse effects of contraception.[7]

Of course, researchers have noted the shock factors. That's why there is a constant search for the "perfect contraceptive"—one that is 100 percent free of all health hazards and side effects, is reversible in 100 percent of all cases, doesn't interfere in any way whatsoever with the act of intercourse, *and* has a 100 percent theoretical *and* use-effectiveness rate.

Some of the ideas developed for the near or far future include contraceptive skin implants, contraceptive bracelets for cutaneous absorption of hormones, "morning-after" abortifacients, the Male Pill, antisperm drugs, and contraceptive vaccinations.

But if we have learned anything at all from our past experience with artificial methods, it is this: *as the effectiveness rates of artificial birth control methods rise, the shock factors also seem to rise.* And in all the really effective artificial methods—the Pill, the IUD, vasectomy, female sterilization—*one* partner absorbs *all* of the shock, although (presumably) both participate in the pleasures.

So why is artificial birth control such a frustrating and difficult feat? Why is it so complicated and, when really effective, apparently so dangerous?

For this reason: at its core, contraception is a fight against nature. Our experience over the past few years has merely shown us that we can attempt to fight nature, but only with consequences.

Does this mean that we can never have effective, hazard-free birth control? That there is no answer?

Happily, no.

In the past few years serious research on fertility awareness has begun to offer men and women a far better family planning alternative. For the first time in history it is possible to practice effective birth control without drugs, without wearing devices, and without ever surrendering to surgery. Consequently, there is no health hazard, no interference with the act of intercourse; and no question whatsoever about irreversibility. In fact, natural family planning can be used *either* to achieve *or* to avoid pregnancy.

Only natural family planning—fertility awareness—demands that you develop an important degree of *self*-awareness, both individually and as a couple. Using these methods, you will learn more about your body, your sexual attitudes, your emotions, your interpersonal relationship with your mate, and your feelings about love.

But this learning process must begin at square one: understanding how male and female bodies cooperate to bring a child into existence.

3

How Male and Female Bodies Cooperate to Conceive a Child

If you ever view sperm cells under magnification, you will see that they resemble tiny tadpoles. Once they are in the female reproductive tract, their tails whip back and forth with astonishing speed, propelling them toward the egg. Upon arrival, the sperm seem to bombard the giant egg, which is 100,000 times bigger. Each sperm has only one mission: acceptance and entry deep into the egg cell nucleus.

And only one will succeed.

Why is one sperm successful and the others not? We don't know. A mysterious process of selection or attraction seems to be at work; what it is remains one of nature's secrets.

But we do know this: when the nuclei of the sperm cell and egg cell interact, something remarkable happens. There comes a moment—after twenty minutes to perhaps an hour or so—when there are no longer two separate entities, a sperm and an egg. Rather, a unique, single-celled human being exists. Some of the original egg cell remains, but the new being has an entirely distinctive structure and identity.

Information exchange. As the merging of the egg and

sperm cells occurs, the genetic information carried in the nucleus of each cell is shared and exchanged. There are approximately 20,000 bits of information in *each* nucleus, and some scientists suspect that there are considerably more.

In one sense, these pieces of information work a little like our alphabet. By combining and recombining the twenty-six letters, all the books, magazines, pamphlets, newspapers, in the English language have been written. If you take into account all the other languages that use the same alphabet, you can't help but be aware of how incredibly rich and varied our twenty-six-letter alphabet is.

And so, too, is the genetic information—the combined 40,000 information bits—that fuses between the nuclei of the two cells. The intricate combinations produce a new individual unlike any other human being who has ever lived—or ever *will* live.

Will this new person have blue or brown eyes? What about hair color? Red? Blond? Black? Or brown? That information comes together at the time of conception. So does information about height and the tendency to be lean or heavy-boned.

Psychological, mental, and temperamental tendencies are probably fused at this time, too. Perhaps the baby will have an easygoing temperament; maybe he or she will have a fiery, tempestuous nature. It's all a mystery, one that will gradually unfold over the years and decades of development following that special moment: conception.

Conception is an example at its most splendid of profound cooperation in nature. Two, male and female, are absolutely essential for the one, male *or* female, to exist.

Conception is also two things at once: the beginning of a new life, and the culmination of certain physical changes and activities in the male and female bodies that make the new life possible.

And it's all of a piece: the conception of your baby

is involved with the changes you must go through. It's enmeshed with the reality of your body, the reality of your spouse's body, and your combined fertility. So while the rest of this chapter may merely seem to be about the male and female bodies, it is really about much more than that. This chapter is about the beginning of life.

The Man's Essential Contribution

From the time of puberty until the day he dies, the male is always potentially fertile. Indeed, his reproductive decades can stretch for forty, fifty, sixty years, and even longer.

How is it that the man's organs can work so constantly, so continuously? How *is* it that men are always fertile?

Male organs. Male external genitals—the penis and the scrotum, the saclike structure suspended beneath the penis—are clearly differentiated and readily visible. Inside the scrotum there are two plum-sized structures called testicles. One specialized group of cells within the testicles produces the immature sperm and another group of specialized cells produces the masculinizing hormone, testosterone. This hormone is responsible for facial and body (including pubic) hair, voice change, and the awakening of sexual interest in the male.

Testosterone is absorbed directly into the bloodstream from the testicular manufacturing site. But the sperm cells, which take about a month to manufacture, follow a well-designated path upon emerging from the testicles.

Sperm cell development. First, the immature sperm pass upward through the epididymis. This can take anywhere from two weeks to a month. But a slow passage is important because it gives the sperm time to mature.

If the male remains continent for a long period of

time, the sperm cells that have completed their journey are stored in the ducts and the epididymis. These cells don't remain there indefinitely; new sperm cells are constantly being produced and mature sperm are removed periodically, even daily.

Assuring a fresh sperm supply. One way to rid the body of older sperm is the phenomenon of the involuntary orgasm: the so-called wet dream or nocturnal emission. But even without an involuntary ejaculation, nature has another way of removing aging sperm: leaking them out in the urine. This "leakage" seems to be a continuous process, since sperm are usually found in the urine of normally fertile men.

In most cases (assuming an ongoing genital relationship) most of the sperm leaves the male as a result of the orgasmic involuntary muscle contractions produced during intercourse. At this time the sperm becomes mixed with other fluids in accessory glands, especially the prostate and the seminal vesicles. The term used for the product of this mixture is semen.

Effects of intercourse. The ejaculation during genital intercourse carries the sperm from the male tract into the female tract. Gradually, over a period of hours, these fluids drain out of the vagina. Most of the time tens of millions of sperm cells die within hours in the vagina. There is one exception: there is a phase in every woman's cycle during which sperm cells are nourished and kept viable for several days within the woman's reproductive tract. But understanding this survival mechanism requires a consideration of female physiology.

The Woman's Essential Contribution

A diagram of a woman's reproductive organs shows a uterus shaped like an upside-down pear flanked on each side by an ovary. In addition, a tube leads from each ovary to the uterus. The bottom of the uterus, the cervix, opens into the vagina—the canal that receives the penis during intercourse.

How conception occurs. After ejaculation, the sperm travel upward from the vaginal canal, through the cervix and the uterus and into the tubes. If ovulation has occurred, one egg (occasionally more) is normally released from one of the ovaries and begins to travel down the Fallopian tube. If some of the sperm cells have succeeded in traveling as far as the tubes, the egg may join with one to create a new individual. But if no sperm are present and no conception takes place, the egg disintegrates. Egg degeneration usually ends within twenty-four hours after ovulation. Thus, *a woman is capable of becoming pregnant only within twenty-four hours of the day she ovulates —not later, not before.*

The menstrual period. If conception does not take place, the uterine lining that had been preparing for that possibility—in effect, creating a biological cradle to hold the pre-natal child—is sloughed off. This is menstruation.

Menstruation usually occurs between twelve and sixteen days after ovulation, although for a very small percentage of women it can occur in as few as four to nine days after ovulation. In others, it may be as long as eighteen, nineteen, twenty days or more after ovulation. While the time span between ovulation and menstruation is quite constant for most women, the time that elapses from menstruation to menstruation is not.

How ovulation occurs. Each woman has an internal "fertility trigger" located in her brain, in the tiny pituitary gland found at its base. This gland emits special hormones, including one that stimulates the growth and development of the ovarian follicle containing the egg. It's called the follicle-stimulating hormone—FSH for short.

Curiously, the length of time it takes for FSH to initiate the active ripening of the follicle—and therefore the egg—can be highly variable and unpredictable. It can take a week, it can take months. But once the amount of FSH released into the body reaches a special "threshold" level, things move quickly *and predictably.*

Within five days, a special group of ovarian follicles that contain eggs are stimulated into active maturation. One of the marks of this stimulation is the secretion of estradiol, the major estrogenic hormone that enters the bloodstream from the follicle and travels up to the pituitary. Its appearance signals the pituitary that the follicle is stimulated.

Once this signal is received, the gland immediately cuts back on FSH production so that no competing follicles can ripen. Then it sends out a different hormone, the luteinizing hormone (LH). This hormone boosts the follicle into the final stage that culminates in its rupture and the release of the egg—the event known as ovulation.

Perfect timing. But here is the fascinating part: according to Thomas W. Hilgers, M.D., assistant professor of obstetrics and gynecology at Creighton University School of Medicine in Omaha, Nebraska, it is only in the last few hours before the follicle ruptures that the major events of maturation occur for the egg. Consequently, it's irrelevant how long any particular cycle lasts. In fact, virtually all the eggs in the ovaries are present *before* a woman is born, from about the tenth week of her fetal development. *The essential matter is proper maturation.* Since this takes place only after FSH production has been cut and LH has entered the bloodstream, and within a very short but well-defined time period, the egg that is ovulated always emerges at the absolutely perfect point of its development—when it's ripe for conception.

Thus, nature has designed both sperm cells and egg cells to emerge at the perfect time—at their peak of maturation—to maximize the possibility of conception.

Achieving conception. This brings us to another

question: if the egg survives less than twenty-four hours out of each cycle, how is it possible to become pregnant more easily than not? How likely is it to time intercourse precisely for pregnancy to occur?

Some mammals—rabbits and ferrets are two examples —ovulate in response to copulation, but this type of ovulation is *not* the human pattern. Instead, nature has a way of "stretching out" a woman's fertile phase: sperm are kept alive for a number of days in the female tract, but *only* during the time in her cycle when the woman is about to ovulate. In this way, fewer acts of intercourse are as likely to lead to conception as numerous acts.

Indeed, this is one of nature's most fascinating stratagems to insure that the human species survives. It's the cornerstone of all modern, scientific natural family planning methods. But how exactly does it work? What is its mechanism?

Vaginal secretions. Most of the time a woman's vaginal secretions are acidic and actively hostile to sperm. This insures against the possibility of sperm living—and aging —in the woman's reproductive tract. But if any sperm are particularly plucky and actually withstand the acid environment, nature provides a second, more effective mechanism to insure that sperm won't travel beyond the vaginal canal: the cervical mucus barrier.

The mucus barrier. Before the ovulation phase begins and immediately after it has ended, the cervical mucus secretions as seen through a scanning electron microscope show a dense maze of tight-knit, meshlike formations. Sperm cells cannot penetrate this maze. But matters change considerably as the time of ovulation approaches.

The gateway. Under a scanning electron microscope, the mucus pattern at the time of ovulation is no longer a maze. Instead, about five days prior to the event, the mucus begins to look like beautiful, crystalline ferns. The little mucus strands no longer "crosshatch" against each other, cutting off possible travel routes for the sperm cells. Instead, the strands arrange themselves in a parallel-type formation, becoming, in effect, a gateway—forming an "entry-type" mucus that does more than just ease sperm penetration. *Entry-type mucus actively enhances sperm cell penetration* through the cervix.

This dramatic mucus change is a result of hormone activity. As follicular activity enters its final stages before ovulation, increasing amounts of estrogen are secreted. Estrogen acts on cervical mucus, changing it from a thick, tenacious, gummy mass, hostile to sperm, to an abundant, clear, watery solution that looks and feels like raw egg white. *This* solution is hospitable to sperm cells. Estrogen is responsible for "lifting the barriers" and making the mucus strands parallel just prior to ovulation—the optimum time for conception to occur.

It is in this fashion that a woman's cervical mucus secretions act like a biological valve, a valve that opens and closes in exquisite harmony with each woman's ovulation patterns. The result? Fresh sperm cells and fresh egg cells are assured in human conception.

One in several hundred million. Now perhaps you can begin to understand more completely what a wondrous event your conception was. Nature carefully designed an astonishing array of special biological mechanisms to insure that an egg cell and a sperm cell would be likely to join and interact when both were at their peak.

In your case, for example, only *that* special sperm cell and *that* special egg cell from your parents could have created you. A few moments more—or a few less—and a different sperm cell might have entered the egg nucleus. That arrival would have made an immense difference, one that is truly unfathomable, imponderable. Not only would a different person be living today, but that person could even have been a member of the opposite sex!

Consider, too, this breathtaking fact: if you think of

the numbers of sperm cells at each ejaculation (possibly as many as 500 million) and the numbers of egg cells available for ripening at each ovulation (as many as a half million), you can see why it can truly be said that *you are one in trillions!*

And the same can be said for every child you conceive.

4

How Your Body Tells You That You're Ready to Conceive a Child

At a day-long medical seminar on contraception that I recently attended, I didn't hear the words "man," "husband," "partner," "spouse," more than once for every 500 or so times I heard the words "the woman."

This view is very lopsided because, in actual fact, *fertility is a shared condition.*

Consider this fact: a normal, healthy man is fertile every hour of his life from puberty to death. But without a woman, a man's splendid day-in, day-out, year-in, year-out fertility is completely useless. Even if a man were to have intercourse with a female of normal fertility, conception is still not assured, since most of the time a woman is infertile.

Thus, male production of several millions and more sperm cells is absolutely worthless in the absence of a woman's single, critical contribution: one viable egg cell. And at a certain point within twenty-four hours after the woman has ovulated, a couple *cannot conceive again under any circumstances whatsoever until the beginning of the fertile phase of the next menstrual cycle.*

Then, once the fertile phase has begun, intercourse can lead to conception, the likelihood increasing as the woman nears the time of ovulation. Indeed, even genital contact *without* penile entry into the vagina or without ejaculation may lead to conception once the fertile phase has begun. The reason? There may be enough sperm in the pre-ejaculatory fluids to result in pregnancy. Some researchers believe that penile leakage can result in conception if the fluid comes into contact with a woman's external genitals when she is in the fertile phase of her cycle.

Natural family planning. A normal woman can't conceive twenty-seven out of twenty-eight days of a so-called "typical" menstrual cycle. In other words, from her first menstruation until the onset of menopause some thirty years or more later, a woman won't be able to conceive approximately 97 percent of the time.

But since conception is a joint affair, it is necessary to take into consideration the *couple's* fertility and infertility. If we combine the sperm's estimated (maximum) survival time of five days with the woman's single day of fertility, then *the couple* is infertile approximately 80 percent of the time during the woman's fertile years.

The long infertile phase offers a potentially revolutionary means of natural family planning. If the infertile phase can be accurately identified, for the first time in history a couple who wishes to avoid conception can express love physically *without the use of any form of contraception whatsoever!*

Consider for a moment just how important this can be to you. The natural method that you will learn in this book offers you the opportunity to plan your family without:

- Resorting to powerful drugs,
- Using chemicals,
- Wearing barrier devices,
- Interrupting the sex act,

- Risking a single hazard to life or health,
- Causing any side effects whatsoever, or
- Permanently affecting either partner's fertility.

What's involved in enjoying such benefits? A *couple* must learn to recognize the onset and end of a woman's constantly recurring fertile and infertile phases. In other words, both partners must learn to "read" the female's body in a new and informative way so they can determine just when some of the biologically required "links" essential for conception are temporarily absent, making conception impossible.

Once you know on a *day-by-day basis* whether or not a particular act of intercourse is likely to lead to conception, your "fertility awareness" can then be used however the two of you mutually agree to use it: either to postpone or avoid conception, or to welcome a child into your lives.

It's your choice.

Post-ovulatory Infertility

Table 1 on page 42 shows twelve different menstrual cycles from twelve different women. The first day of menstruation is Day 1 of a new cycle.

You will notice that the length of the ovulatory and the post-ovulatory phases is constant for all twelve women. This is because no matter how long a woman's cycle is—and these cycles range from twenty-six to forty-four days—the ovulatory and post-ovulatory phases remain constant, since menstruation generally occurs about twelve to sixteen days after ovulation.

In contrast, the menstrual/post-menstrual phase is *highly variable* for different women—and it can also vary a few days from cycle to cycle for the same woman. It is the variability in *this* phase that determines the total length of each cycle.

TABLE 1:

MENSTRUAL/POST-MENSTRUAL PHASE	OVULATORY PHASE	POST-OVULATORY PHASE
Couple is infertile	Couple is fertile Conception is likely	Couple is infertile

1 2 3 4 5 6 7 8 9 10 11 12 13 14 15 16 17 18 19 20 21 22 23	24 25 26 27 28 29 30 31 32 33	34 35 36 37 38 39 40 41 42 43 44
1 2 3 4 5 6 7 8 9 10 11 12	13 14 15 16 17 18 19 20 21 22	23 24 25 26 27 28 29 30 31 32 33
1 2 3 4 5 6 7 8 9 10 11 12 13 14 15	16 17 18 19 20 21 22 23 24 25	26 27 28 29 30 31 32 33 34 35 36
1 2 3 4 5 6 7 8 9 10 11 12 13 14 15 16 17	18 19 20 21 22 23 24 25 26 27	28 29 30 31 32 33 34 35 36 37 38
1 2 3 4 5	6 7 8 9 10 11 12 13 14 15	16 17 18 19 20 21 22 23 24 25 26
1 2 3 4 5 6 7 8 9 10 11 12 13 14 15 16 17 18 19 20 21 22	23 24 25 26 27 28 29 30 31 32	33 34 35 36 37 38 39 40 41 42 43
1 2 3 4 5 6	7 8 9 10 11 12 13 14 15 16	17 18 19 20 21 22 23 24 25 26 27
1 2 3 4 5 6 7 8	9 10 11 12 13 14 15 16 17 18	19 20 21 22 23 24 25 26 27 28 29
1 2 3 4 5 6 7 8 9 10 11 12 13 14	15 16 17 18 19 20 21 22 23 24	25 26 27 28 29 30 31 32 33 34 35
1 2 3 4 5 6 7 8 9	10 11 12 13 14 15 16 17 18 19	20 21 22 23 24 25 26 27 28 29 30
1 2 3 4 5 6 7 8 9 10 11 12 13	14 15 16 17 18 19 20 21 22 23	24 25 26 27 28 29 30 31 32 33 34
1 2 3 4 5 6 7 8 9 10 11 12 13 14 15 16	17 18 19 20 21 22 23 24 25 26	27 28 29 30 31 32 33 34 35 36 37

The length of the menstrual/post-menstrual phase is highly variable for different women and can even vary from cycle to cycle for the same woman. It is the variability in this phase that determines the total length of each cycle; the lengths of the ovulatory and post-ovulatory phases remain highly constant for all women.

42

While we usually think of the menstrual/post-menstrual phase as the beginning of a new cycle, note that it is also a *continuation* of the post-ovulatory phase. You can see this quite readily by looking at Table 2 on page 44 where the cycle is drawn as a circle. Note that the couple's infertility is continuous through the post-ovulatory and the menstrual/post-menstrual phases.

It is important to note this continuous phase of infertility because study after study has shown that there is absolutely no chance for conception to occur once a woman has entered the post-ovulatory phase of her cycle.[1] Conception becomes likely only when she enters the ovulatory phase of the *succeeding* cycle, when the cervical mucus secretions change into a solution that not only is hospitable to sperm but actually aids their survival.

Determining the infertile time. One method gives a couple the highest possible assurance that the post-ovulatory infertile phase has begun. Thus, it offers reliability equivalent to the Pill or tubal sterilization. The method? It's a simple matter of monitoring a woman's waking temperatures.

Every woman's waking temperatures change throughout her cycle. They are lower at the beginning of the cycle; they're about a half a degree higher during the last two weeks. *When a woman's waking temperatures are high, she is infertile.* Pregnancy cannot take place once a woman has entered the high temperature phase of the cycle.

Explaining your temperature rise. Why does this temperature rise occur? What causes it?

After the egg cell is released, the ovarian follicle begins to manufacture the hormone *progesterone*. Progesterone does three things:

1. Causes a woman's basal body waking temperature to rise;

TABLE 2

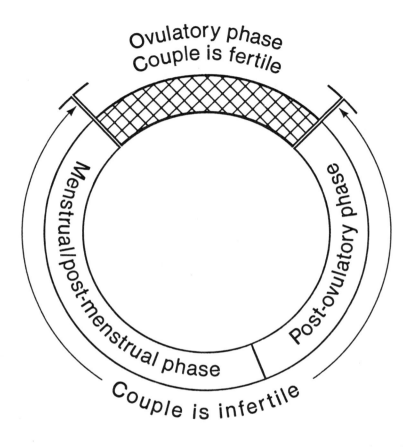

The couple's infertility is continuous from the beginning of the post-ovulatory phase through the end of the menstrual/post-menstrual phase.

2. Dries up cervical mucus;
3. Suppresses all further ovulations for the rest of the cycle.*

But please recognize that you cannot pinpoint the day of ovulation from a review of your temperatures. *The only thing temperatures can tell you is when your infertile time has definitely begun.* Acts of intercourse that take place during the infertile phase cannot result in conception. (Note: you will receive specific instructions on charting temperature and all fertility signs in Part II of this book, beginning on page 113.

Research results. Just how reliable is the so-called temperature method? One study by Dr. Gerhard Doering (West Germany) followed 307 couples over 11,352 cycles —an average of almost three years' participation per couple. There was a total of eight unplanned pregnancies—*not one of which occurred after a third high temperature had been properly recorded.* Thus, Doering's study showed 100 percent reliability for the method when intercourse takes place *after* the third high temperature is recorded.[2]

Dr. John Marshall, a participant in the June, 1966, Geneva scientific group meeting on the biology of fertility control by periodic abstinence, has also done work on post-ovulatory infertility. He reports that in his study in England of 5,013 cycles in which the dates of intercourse were known, "there was not a single instance of conception

---

* Progesterone has another essential task if conception takes place: it helps prepare the uterine lining for the implantation of a tiny embryo. If conception has occurred in that particular cycle, the follicle will continue to produce progesterone to sustain the pregnancy.

In fact, one way of discovering if you are pregnant even before the doctor can tell is to note whether the high level of progesterone is sustained in your body for seven days beyond the expected beginning of the menstrual period. So if your waking temperature remains elevated for a full week beyond its usual elevated duration, you have 99 percent assurance that pregnancy has been achieved.

occurring when intercourse had been confined to the phase after three temperatures at the higher level had been recorded."[3]

Perhaps you can understand why the well-known population and family planning expert associated with the Population Council, Christopher Tietze, M.D., has ranked this natural method with the combination Pill and surgical sterilization as one of the most reliable birth control measures of all. It outranks both the mini-Pill and the IUD in effectiveness.[4]

Although Dr. Tietze didn't mention the fact, this effectiveness is possible without a single hazard to your health or your fertility.

Menstrual/Post-Menstrual Infertility

Since you cannot conceive after an indisputable temperature rise has been established, all the days between confirmation of the rise and the beginning of the following menstruation (menses) are absolutely infertile. Indeed, if you look at Table 2 on page 44, you will note the continuation of infertility through the beginning of the menstrual phase.

But there's a new question: how long does infertility last in the menstrual/post-menstrual phase? How long can the couple have relations during this phase without conception taking place?

Continuation of infertility. The couple remains infertile during the menstrual/post-menstrual phase for an indeterminate length of time. The single most important fertility indicator is the development and change in a woman's cervical mucus secretions. (Note: the sustained high temperature only reflects *the onset of infertility*.) Indeed, the development of cervical mucus has recently been recognized to be so important an index of the beginning of the fertile phase that some experienced couples rely solely on it to determine fertility and infertility. The Ovulation Method of natural family planning relies exclusively on this indicator.

There is a sound reason for this reliance, of course. As we saw previously, during the ovulatory phase the cervical mucus changes in response to the increasing estrogen in a woman's body. Chemically, these secretions become less acidic (hostile to sperm) and more alkaline (hospitable to sperm). But these secretions also change *structurally*.

Cervical mucus changes. If you could look at the cervical secretions under a microscope, you would discover that as ovulation approaches, the little mucus strands begin to arrange themselves in a parallel formation. The likelihood of conception increases if a couple has genital contact, including sexual relations, nearer the actual time of ovulation because sperm cells have a greater likelihood of passing through this parallel formation. *You can monitor these changes in your cervical secretions without the use of a microscope or knowledge of the chemical composition of the mucus.*

What to look for. The changes in mucus have been recognized since the late 1930s and early 1940s by physicians working with infertile couples. In the 1960s two Australian physicians—a husband and wife, Drs. John and Evelyn Billings—realized that women could learn to monitor the changes in their mucus secretions just from observation of the vulva, the external female genital area.

The mucus changes follow one another in a regular, *unfolding* pattern and do *not* depend on cyclic regularity. You will observe these changes whether your cycles are long or short. The only difference is that beginning mucus changes may be delayed or intermittent, ultimately determining the "cycle length."

Once you become alert to the changes—and their

meaning in terms of fertility—you will know whether a specific act of intercourse can lead to conception in a new menstrual cycle.

What should you be looking for?

The infertile dry days. Let's assume your menstrual bleeding ended after about four or five days. The vagina itself will be moist, but externally there is a distinct sensation of dryness. You may notice a feeling of mild itchiness around the vaginal entrance. Perhaps a little additional estrogen is entering your system, but at this point there's not enough to create any real changes in the cervical mucus—at least, not any changes you can detect. Thus, there will usually be a handful of so-called dry days.

You are infertile during the dry days. Acts of intercourse will not lead to conception when the vagina is without mucus.

The Fertile Ovulatory Phase

Assuming you don't have short cycles in which the ovulatory phase immediately follows the menstrual bleeding, you will notice mucus for the first time sometime after the dry days have passed. The onset of mucus marks the possible beginning of the ovulatory phase.

Sticky, tacky mucus. The first mucus you see will probably be of a special consistency. Perhaps the best way to explain it is to remind you of school days when you sometimes used a white paste that was sticky and tacky. The first mucus you observe may remind you of that paste.

You won't have to go searching for the mucus since it's usually readily detectable near the vaginal opening. Sticky, tacky mucus is usually opaque white or yellow. If you place this mucus between your thumb and forefinger, you'll notice that it makes tiny little peaks when you separate the fingers. The mucus is also rather thick and will hold its shape quite well.

Microscopically and chemically, the sticky, tacky mucus is still a barrier to sperm. However, the cervical mucus secretions can change over a period of hours (in less than a half-day or so) so that the microscopic strands start to move in a parallel position. Microscopic "gateways" will open, offering some possibility for the sperm to travel up through the cervix toward the Fallopian tubes. Since this change can be rapid, consider yourselves fertile on any day you notice this type of mucus as well as on three full days that follow its cessation. If there is no mucus on the fourth day, you are infertile that evening. (Note: specific charting instructions are detailed in Part II of this book, beginning on page 113.)

Thin, watery, cloudy mucus. When the cervical secretions become thin, watery, possibly milky, and rather cloudy-looking in appearance—like smooth, creamy hand lotion—your body may be preparing for ovulation. You could conceive a child!

This type of mucus may also look somewhat translucent whether it's yellow or white in color. You may sometimes notice that it appears to be a little bit red, pink, or brown. This is caused by spotting and is perfectly normal for many women. As long as the spotting or bleeding is accompanied by developing mucus, it should not concern you.

The thin, watery, or cloudy mucus is detectable on the external genitals just by a feeling of wetness that was previously absent. Also, if you get a dab of the mucus between two fingers and draw the fingers apart, it won't make little peaks; it will remain smooth on both fingers like a dab of creamy hand lotion.

Since sperm can survive in this favorable mucus environment, you're fertile. *If you don't wish to conceive during this cycle, you must both agree to abstain completely from all genital contact, including intercourse, when you feel any sensation of wetness, or if your mucus appears to be thin, watery, creamy, cloudy-looking, or translucent.* The duration of this type of mucus is highly variable for each woman. It could last a day or two or several days. Occasionally, the mucus reverts to the sticky, tacky consistency for a day or more. However, this change does not alter the fact that the woman's body is in a phase that could result in conception. The couple is fertile; acts of intercourse will probably cause pregnancy.

Slippery, lubricative mucus. When estrogen is highest in your bloodstream (and there's no progesterone, to speak of, circulating in your system yet), the mucus is likely to become extremely profuse. The mucus changes in appearance, too: it looks like raw egg white—completely clear and "glarey" (shiny).

As for *feel* and *quality*, the mucus is much like raw egg white. If you were to take a small amount of this mucus between two fingers, it would feel very slippery. Then if you were to draw the fingers apart, the mucus would stretch at least an inch—or even several inches—until it looked like a long, thin, shimmering thread. The ability of the mucus to be stretched into a thread is an important phenomenon with a special German name: *Spinnbarkeit.*

You are *most* likely to conceive during the days when slippery, lubricative mucus is present. Do *not* engage in either genital contact or acts of intercourse if you do not wish to conceive a child at this time.

The very last day of the slippery, lubricative mucus is known as the "mucus peak."

Does the mucus peak mean that your fertile phase is nearly over? Will you be able to consider yourselves infertile the next day or two?

No, you won't.

You see, at this stage in our knowledge, it is not possible to pinpoint the *exact* moment of ovulation. However, special hormonal measurements indicate that ovulation can sometimes occur as late as three whole days *after* the mucus peak. It may also occur as early as two days before the peak. However, it is impossible to determine the moment of ovulation, even in the laboratory. For this reason, *our major concern is to "bracket" the fertile days.* This bracketing can be readily accomplished. Certainty about the exact time of ovulation cannot.

So the question comes back to this one: when are you infertile again? When can intercourse take place without conception?

Drying-up days. After the mucus peak has passed, a number of dry or drying-up days will usually begin. This is the direct effect of the progesterone's action on the cervical mucus secretions. The estrogen levels may actually be *higher* after ovulation, but they will be *opposed* by the progesterone. The hormone will suppress further ovulations, and at the same time it will cause the mucus to change.

Mucus and temperature signs. How do these two signs relate? Shouldn't the drying up coincide with the temperature rise?

Perhaps it should . . . in *theory.* In reality we are not programmed machines.

According to New York City physician Dr. Edward F. Keefe: "If you have seen or felt lots of slippery, lubricative, raw-egg-white mucus in the past two days, continue to abstain no matter what the temperature chart shows. In other words, don't go by temperature in the face of contradictory mucus signs, nor by mucus in the face of sure low-temperature readings."

Indeed, there is no *fixed* time relationship between the mucus peak and ovulation: variations of several days either way are within the range of normalcy, and guidelines have been devised to take these variations into account.

Dr. Josef Roetzer has devised what is probably the

easiest and most reliable mucus-with-temperature guide-line: *after the cessation of the fertile-time mucus, look for three consecutive high temperatures above the highest of six consecutive temperatures just before the rise begins. The last of the three temperatures must be 0.4° higher than the highest of those six lower temperatures.*

In other words, *after* the mucus peak, when the drying up begins—and *only* after it begins—should you rely on the third of the high temperatures before considering yourselves infertile. Sometimes you may notice one or more days of mucus well after the peak, even after the third high temperature has been recorded. This is a transitory phenomenon. It sometimes occurs, but you can consider yourselves infertile provided you followed the guidelines.

Infertility in the new cycle. Dr. Roetzer has seen no pregnancies from an act of intercourse on Day 5 of a new cycle *following a sustained temperature rise in the previous cycle.* Therefore, once the third high temperature has been recorded after the cessation of mucus, a couple is considered infertile from 8:00 P.M. of that day through and including the evening of the fifth day of the new cycle.[5]

A couple could be fertile on Day 6 of the new menstrual cycle. The possibility is so small that Dr. Roetzer considers the sixth day infertile for all, including couples whose cycles are shorter than twenty-six days.* "Theoretically, it seems almost impossible that an intercourse on the sixth day of a genuine cycle should result in a conception," reports Dr. Roetzer.[6] Dr. Roetzer has observed only one Day 6 pregnancy in a study of 200 women with over 6,000 doctor-supervised cycles. This particular Day 6

---

* Some authorities hold that any woman who ever experiences cycles shorter than twenty-two days should consider the sixth cycle day to be a fertile day.

pregnancy occurred to a couple with a history of short, 22- to 27-day cycles. Thus, the reliability factor for Day 6 infertility is considered to be 99.8 percent at this writing. This is an overall figure for all couples with all kinds of cycle lengths.

Dr. Roetzer has no statistics for the fertility of Day 7 per se, but he reports that it can be fertile for some couples, particularly those who ever experience cycles 27 days or shorter. *By Day 7 you should be very alert to possible mucus.*

Day 8 is definitely in the fertile range for couples who experience cycle lengths of at least 28 days.

Effectiveness. Are Dr. Roetzer's guidelines reliable? Can you count on high effectiveness in avoiding pregnancy?

You can.

In a study conducted by Dr. Roetzer, 491 couples of previously proven fertility followed all guidelines over 17,026 cycles. Only twelve surprise pregnancies were recorded.

What's more impressive is this fact: this is an *overall use-effectiveness figure,* not a "theoretical" or "biological" effectiveness figure.[7] Real couples, actual users—including casual users and careless ones—were included in the study.

If you want to convert those twelve surprise pregnancies to a method-effectiveness rate (which is easier to deal with for comparative purposes), this is a method with a use-effectiveness rate of 99.2 percent.

This is also a method that is 100 percent free of any risk to your health or future fertility.

Movement of the Cervix

For a long time researchers have hoped to develop a simple, easy-to-use biological test system to let a woman know when ovulation is about to occur or is actually occurring. But as often happens in man's attempts to outwit nature, nature beat us.

As it turns out, every woman carries her own built-in biological test system: her cervix. Any woman can feel the cervix, the lower part of the uterus, simply by inserting a finger up into the vagina. If you've ever wondered why a tampon can only go so far up into the vagina, it's because it's stopped by the closed upper portion of the vagina—the cervix. This part of a woman's internal organs is round, with a small opening in the middle, like a dimple.

The sperm pass up into the uterus through this cervical opening during the ovulatory phase. If no sperm have passed—or if sperm have passed but conception doesn't take place—then the menstrual bleeding will leave the uterus through the cervix and pass out of the body through the vagina.

Fertility indicator. The cervix is significant in terms of your fertility awareness. Depending on where you are in your cycle, the cervix exhibits marked changes. Dr. Edward F. Keefe, the first doctor to have systematically studied and published papers about the phenomenon of the rising cervix during the ovulatory phase, candidly admits that he first learned about the phenomenon from his patients. He instructed them to "milk the cervix" if they had difficulty detecting mucus. But as the time of ovulation approached, the women experienced difficulty reaching the cervix. Yet when the women were infertile, there was no problem at all.

When Dr. Keefe heard this reaction from enough women, he recognized that this could be a significant factor in determining fertility.

Cervical changes. It appears that the cervix is responsive to the contraction and extension of ligaments that hold it "in place." These ligaments are, in turn, responsive to the amount of estrogen and progesterone in a woman's body.

As more and more estrogen enters a woman's bloodstream in the pre-ovulatory phase, the estrogens contract the cervical supports at the base of the broad ligaments. Result? Over a period of days it becomes harder and harder for a woman to reach her cervix, since it's being progressively drawn *up* into the vagina as much as an inch or more. But around the time of ovulation, when the follicle or the ruptured follicle begins to release progesterone into the woman's bloodstream, the ligaments relax. Then the cervix seems to descend into the vagina, where it's again within easy reach.

Besides the "up and away" cervical movement, there is another change that you will be able to detect. The cervix will change from being firm, like the tip of your nose, to being soft, spongy, and sometimes rubbery. It will feel yielding and soft, like your lips.

Again, these changes parallel the hormonal fluctuations in the body. When there's more progesterone, the cervix is firm. But as more estrogen enters the bloodstream, the cervix softens and loses its firmness completely. And that, of course, is the time when you are getting close to, or are actually at, the day of ovulation.

Once the body's progesterone levels begin to rise, the cervix progressively lowers into the vagina and becomes firm to the touch within days.

There's another change: the cervical opening, known as the *os* (Latin for "mouth") really *opens* at the time of ovulation. If you have had a child, it may even be possible for you to introduce a fingertip into the os at this time. During the infertile phase, when there's a high level of progesterone in the system, the os is closed tightly and is sometimes "plugged" with the sticky, tacky mucus that makes the passage resolutely impenetrable to sperm.

Noting the cervical changes can be very helpful if you're confused about mucus signs, since it allows you to check one sign against another. You will usually find coincidence between the mucus changes and the cervical movement if you're ovulating normally.

Recognizing the changes. Of all the signs of fertility, this one is the hardest to recognize, especially in the beginning when it's most subjective. "I couldn't figure it out at first," said one woman. "Was the cervix higher? Was it softer? I just wasn't sure. It took me three months before I got the hang of it."

Most women need to go through several cycles, at least three or four, before they can readily detect the cervical changes. No woman feels at home monitoring the changes in the first two cycles.

Is the cervical sign useful? Does it really help a couple evaluate their fertility?

Dr. Keefe has found that about 25 percent of those he has worked with have ranked the cervical changes as one of the most important, easily detectable signs of ovulation. This group used it readily to decide about fertility or infertility on a particular day.

On the other hand, another 25 percent found the cervical sign to be less valuable than the other fertility indicators. They tended to depend on other signs even though they were aware of the "biological test system" they carried around in their bodies day in and day out.[8]

Other Fertility Indicators

The mucus changes, cervical changes, and temperature shift are all standard fertility/infertility indicators for women. This summary is useful:

MENSTRUAL/POST–MENSTRUAL PHASE: *The couple is infertile. Acts of intercourse will not cause pregnancy.*

Temperature: Low

Mucus: Dry days (no fertile-time mucus)

Cervix: Closed, low, and firm

Duration of phase: Highly variable, lasting from 5
days to many weeks.

OVULATORY PHASE: *The couple is fertile; conception is likely. If pregnancy is not desired, avoid intercourse or genital-genital contact.*

Temperature: Rising

Mucus: Sticky, tacky mucus developing into fertile-
time (slippery, lubricative) mucus, then re-
verting back to sticky-tacky mucus and/or
disappearing.

Cervix: Open, high, and soft

Duration of phase: Somewhat variable, but usually
lasts about seven to eleven days.
Still, this phase may "last" longer
in some cases.

POST–OVULATORY PHASE: *Couple is infertile.
Acts of intercourse will not result in pregnancy.*

Temperature: High

Mucus: Dry (no fertile-time mucus)

Cervix: Closed, low, and firm

Duration of phase: Least variable phase of the cycle.
It usually lasts about 10 to 15
days for 90 percent of all women.

The three major signs of fertility are present in all
women. Each woman, however, is unique and can experience signs of fertility that are distinctly her own.

For example, some women experience breast tenderness around the time of ovulation. Others feel mild discomfort, even pain, for two to nine days around the time
they ovulate. Sometimes the pain is so distinct that a
woman can tell which ovary—left or right—is releasing the
egg.

The following is a listing of ovulatory signs that have
been reported by some women. Perhaps you share one or
two:

- Bloating (shoes feel tight; rings don't fit)
- Insomnia
- Acne
- Chills
- Cold hands and feet
- Mood changes (depression, exuberance, or swings between both)
- Gum bleeding
- Greasy hair
- Spotting
- Heavy feeling or dull ache low in the pelvic area at the level of the vulva

Men sometimes report that they can detect the couple's time of fertility by changes in the wife's mood and/ or by certain physical changes in her body. These are some of the female bodily changes that have been noted by husbands:

- Skin feels smoother
- Skin surface is noticeably warmer
- Change in the color of the vulva (female external genitals)

Fertility Awareness

Awareness of fertility offers a woman—and a couple —a powerful tool for self-understanding. It can sometimes improve relations, as it did for this couple:

My wife gets irritable for a day or two around the time she ovulates. Since I keep the charts, I know in advance when to expect this. We still have fights, but they're quick, two-minute things. We both know what's behind the flare-up.

Another young couple came to a new understanding about the wife's sexual feelings:

> A few days before menstruation I feel achey and uncomfortable—we both understood that and we never had intercourse. However, there were many other days when I was totally uninterested. It seemed as if I were always making excuses to pass up love-making. We were both beginning to wonder if it were something psychological.
>
> After learning the fertility signs, we realized that I feel uncomfortable during the ovulatory phase. Since I have short cycles—twenty-three to twenty-five days—there are many days per cycle when I have no interest in intercourse.
>
> This awareness has lifted a burden for both of us. We now know our problem was physiological—not psychological. Today we're very comfortable with each other sexually.

Health anxiety relief. Many women who had experienced uncomfortable ovulatory signs thought they signaled health problems. So it was a relief for one woman to learn that the discomfort she felt again and again was ovulatory pain—not the first tentative signs of an impending appendicitis attack. Another woman felt mild disturbances in the general area of her abdomen. Another worry laid to rest: she had suspected the onset of bleeding ulcers.

Peace of mind. Use of natural family planning can offer relief in unexpected ways. This mother's experience is illuminating:

> One time while we were still using contraceptives, my period was two and a half weeks late. Naturally, I

suspected pregnancy. Unfortunately, I had taken strong medication a few weeks before when I'd had a bad flu. So for almost three weeks I worried myself sick: did my medication hurt a developing fetus? I was beside myself until the day menstruation finally began.

But it wasn't until just a few weeks ago that I realized just how different things can be with NFP. My son's leg had to be X-rayed. The technician was reluctant to allow me to go into the room with my eighteen-month-old baby, since I could possibly be pregnant. I just couldn't let my baby go in the room all by himself! I was able to assure the man that I was not pregnant. But before NFP I would have been uncertain and would have taken a chance. Instead, it was a beautiful feeling to be able to enter that room with complete peace of mind.

Fertility awareness gives me the complete control over my reproductive life that I never had before.

Self-awareness. A working woman told me that she takes advantage of the ebb and flow of her cycle to do her job. Tasks requiring sustained concentration and attention—researching and writing major company reports—are scheduled for the first few days of a new cycle and during her ovulatory phases. She has learned that concentration is best at those times.

In contrast, this woman reports a slight elevation of tension a few days before her menstrual flow begins. Sustained concentration is more difficult. Therefore, these days are reserved for getting rid of nuisance jobs—sending short letters and memos, checking certain facts and figures to be used in a future presentation, and the like.

A computer softwares saleswoman is highly irregular and suffers from cramping, nausea, and physical distress when menstruation begins. This woman keeps track of only one fertility sign: her mucus peak. Reason? She knows that menstruation will follow thirteen days later. Now she never schedules either a flight or an appointment with an important customer on Day 1 of a new cycle. This was never possible before she learned to recognize her fertility signs.

Of course, fertility awareness is helpful in other areas besides the work place. A mother of seven recognized that she was too lenient with the children during her ovulatory phases (*"nothing* bothers me then"). She works at striking a balance throughout her cycle.

Another woman's yearning for a baby was sometimes overwhelming. When she learned NFP, she recognized when those "times" occurred: three or four days during her ovulatory phases.

The couple had very serious, urgent reasons for avoiding pregnancy. "But I'm sure that I would have gone ahead with a pregnancy if we had used contraceptives," she reported. "I don't think that I would have been able to help myself." Instead, the recognition that her acute longing for a baby had a hormonal basis—and would pass with the ending of her ovulatory phase—made it far easier to cope with pregnancy avoidance. There was an unexpected bonus: "My husband now understands what's happening and helps me get through the days when I ache for another little one. He has also developed some lovely ways of making me feel sexually attractive without allowing me to seduce him. I never expected so much consideration from him and I *never* thought of him as sensitive —but he is."

Medical advantages. Many doctors report medical advantages to fertility awareness. "The first time I had a woman come into my office and tell me that she was twenty-two days pregnant was a real eye-opener to me," a Connecticut physician reported. "I now find that NFP mothers come in for pre-natal care much sooner than any other group of women."

Another advantage: Knowing the time of conception can help a doctor manage a difficult pregnancy if complications develop. Sometimes the age of the fetus determines which procedures can or cannot be risked. Pregnancy aside, women often report vaginal infections almost as soon as they develop. The temporarily confused mucus sign triggers the woman's alertness, bringing her in for a medical examination much sooner. In a few cases, learners have been referred to physicians by their teaching couple because the mucus sign indicated possible pathology. More than one case of cervical cancer has been caught in the early curable stage because of NFP awareness.

Where to go from here. The last two chapters have given you an overview of human reproduction, including the signs of fertility. If you want to "put it all together," that is, begin charting, turn directly to page 113 where detailed charting instructions begin.

On the other hand, some couples allow nature to space their first few children. There are important benefits surrounding natural child-spacing through breast-feeding. I urge you to consider this option if you are just beginning or haven't yet completed desired family size. Information can be found beginning on page 199.

Chapter 13 is for couples with certain kinds of infertility problems. The possibility of conception can be enhanced by properly timing acts of intercourse. That chapter begins on page 222.

Finally, there are other aspects of natural family planning that transcend the question of avoiding or planning a pregnancy. In my case, the consideration of these aspects radicalized my view of human sexuality. The next five chapters offer some radical notions for your consideration.

5

Contraception and Natural Family Planning: What the Experts Say

Without abstinence, there is no natural family planning.

Abstinence would appear to be the drawback to natural birth control. *But astonishingly, couple after couple have reported that, while difficult, the required abstinence period has turned out to be another advantage of using natural methods!*

The conclusion was unexpected and surprising, but there had to be something to it. I had interviewed almost 200 men and women in personal, face-to-face interviews and talked to another 45 to 50 individuals by telephone. To learn if the responses would be different with complete anonymity, I sent out approximately 260 six-page, essay-type questionnaires. One hundred fifty-seven were returned. No matter how I sought the information, the overwhelming response was that natural methods were "satisfactory" or "moderately satisfactory" . . . but more often "highly satisfactory." These ratings were made most often by couples who had used artificial methods over a long period of time—predominantly the Pill—so they had something to compare.

Indeed, these couples gave very high ratings to natural family planning—despite the abstinence—and surprisingly low ratings to contraceptives. For example, only

10.6 percent of those who had used contraceptives rated them as "highly satisfactory." In contrast, natural family planning methods were rated "highly satisfactory" by 74.5 percent. On the other end of the scale, 26.1 percent of the respondents considered contraception to be "highly unsatisfactory," but only 1.8 percent of the respondents gave the same low rating to NFP.*

This apparent high satisfaction rate was sustained when the respondents were asked if they would recommend natural family planning to others. Only 1.2 percent reported that they would not make this recommendation, while a smaller percentage (0.6 percent) reported that *usually* they would not recommend the methods to anyone.

In contrast, 89.8 percent of the respondents reported that they would recommend natural family planning to others; 0.6 percent said that they would recommend the methods, but with reservations.

Only 0.6 percent of the respondents left the question unanswered; 7.0 percent were equivocal. In other words, they would recommend the methods sometimes to some couples and not to others.

This high satisfaction rate for natural methods corresponds with other statistical evidence:

Item: A 1969 survey funded by the Nuffield Foundation interviewed 2,179 couples living in Mauritius, a poor island country in the Indian Ocean. The couples had all

---

* In fact, a total of 58.8 percent of the respondents rated contraception as having been either moderately unsatisfactory, unsatisfactory, or highly unsatisfactory, whereas a total of only 4.5 percent of this same group gave NFP such low ratings.

Total positive response to contraception—that is, either moderately satisfactory, satisfactory, or highly satisfactory—was 33.4 percent. In contrast, total positive responses to natural family planning was 93.5 percent, and, as noted before, 74.5 percent actually rated the natural method as "highly satisfactory" (7.3 percent made no evaluation of contraception and 1.8 percent made no evaluation of NFP).
Note: All figures are rounded and thus do not add up to 100 percent.

learned the Temperature Method of natural family planning some seven years previously and researchers wanted to know how many were still practicing this particular variant of NFP. Results: 83 percent were still relying on the Temperature Method seven years later. Only 96 couples (or 4.4 percent) had changed to an artificial method. The rest of the couples either switched to calendar rhythm (2.4 percent), wanted children at the time of the interview (1.2 percent), or no longer had any need for birth control (menopause, separation, etc.).[1]

In comparison, family planning researchers have noted that the dropout rate for any artificial method is as high as *50 percent within the first year!*

Item: A two-year study of approximately 1,000 couples in five countries (United States, Colombia, France, Canada, and Mauritius) conducted by Claude A. Lanctôt, M.D., M.P.H., Frank J. Rice, Ph.D., and Consuelo Garcia-Devesa, Ph.D., under the auspices of Fairfield University in Connecticut showed that only 4.1 percent had abandoned NFP for either an artificial or surgical method during the course of the study.[2]

Item: A study in England of 410 couples followed over two and a quarter years showed that 74 percent of the husbands and 75 percent of the wives felt that the Temperature Method had helped their marriages. (Only 9 percent of the husbands and 8 percent of the wives felt that it had hindered the marital relationship; the rest of the respondents weren't sure.)[3]

Why were satisfaction levels so high? Why were so many couples willing to stick to a method that involves abstinence?

Disequilibrium: Contraception's Equal Partner

One element becomes most apparent in reading psychological literature concerning contraception: there is often an intrinsic disequilibrium whenever artificial methods are used. Recognizing this disequilibrium, some researchers attempt to "tailor" the appropriate contraceptive to the couple, depending on which partner is more or less "responsible."

For example, Dr. Charles H. Debrovner, M.D., clinical associate professor of obstetrics and gynecology at the New York University School of Medicine, suggests that "female-oriented" contraceptives such as the Pill, diaphragm, etc., are suitable if the woman is able to assume responsibility and isn't subordinate to her husband. In contrast, Dr. Debrovner favors "male-oriented" contraception—which boils down to condoms—if the husband is more dominant and the wife is unwilling to take responsibility for contraception.[4]

Dr. Peter Barglow, director of psychiatric residency training at Northwestern University Medical School in Chicago, believes that taking contraception out of the woman's control is "risky." In his opinion, "the only indication for advising a woman to have her partner use the condom is complete inability to use any kind of contraceptive device herself."[5]

Dr. Ruth W. Lidz, who works with Yale University's department of psychiatry, makes no bones about the disequilibrium that contraception can foster in the marital relationship. She points out that when partners have grown up in settings where male/female roles are distinct, the "marital equilibrium" is often upset if the wife handles birth control for the couple. This is especially the case if the man needs to be dominant; he may actually try to interfere with contraception. On the other hand, assumption of family planning responsibility can be upsetting for some women. They become anxious and uneasy, preferring their husbands to "take the responsibility and control."[6]

One example of disequilibrium is expressed by Dr.

Charles V. Ford, adjunct associate professor of psychiatry at the University of California School of Medicine. Dr. Ford writes: "Initially contraceptive choice must include whether or not one wishes to communicate one's intentions to the spouse or the sexual partner."[7] And certainly some modes of birth control are so unilateral (vasectomy, the Pill, tubal ligation) that one *can* insure that pregnancy does not occur without even revealing one's intentions to a spouse or sexual partner. On the other hand, a woman can make a unilateral—and private—decision to abandon use of the Pill to achieve a desired pregnancy.

What couples say. That contraception tends to engender at least mild disequilibrium came through in reading the questionnaires. A husband whose wife had been on the Pill described what he liked about it: "I didn't have to think."

Another husband reported that the couple had used the condom before switching to natural methods. But his wife also reported use of the diaphragm, foam, and the Pill. Could it be that the wife had been at least partially unwilling to "communicate her intentions" to her husband? But after thoughtfully reviewing both the question and its answer, I understood the disparity in their answers. The question read: "Were you using any birth control methods (including rhythm or coitus interruptus) prior to changing to NFP? If so, which method (or methods) did you use and for how long?" The man's answer was a model of precision: *he* had used the condom—a perfectly adequate response when "you" in the question is taken as a singular pronoun.

At heart, contraception is a singular affair.

Minor disequilibrium. The disequilibrium is not always flagrant or persistent. Sometimes it only seems to "flare up" under certain circumstances. For one woman, a vacation experience caused a minor flare:

I didn't plan too well. Anyway, I ran out of contraceptive jelly for my diaphragm. My husband became
extremely annoyed and said to me, "You should have
been better prepared." What he meant was that *I*
should have been better prepared to provide for *his*
pleasure, and *he* shouldn't have to worry about a
thing.

A woman with a surprise mini-Pill pregnancy reported a milder version of this disequilibrium:

Once we got over our bolt-out-of-the-blue aston-
ishment, my husband and I were actually rather
pleased that I was pregnant. Still, I remember that
when we first got the report I was left with a feeling
that *I* had failed at something that was *my* job.

For some couples, the use of artificial methods may
be symptomatic of deeper problems of manipulation, control, and unequal commitment. The following story from
a woman now separated from her second husband would
seem a case in point:

I once sat Jack down and really explained to him
how much I wanted *us* to have a baby, the two of us.
He felt that since we each had children from previous marriages, there was no reason to have any
more. I talked to him for nearly three hours, trying
to explain to him exactly how much it meant to me.
I didn't think he understood a word I said. But I was
wrong.
    One thing changed after that long talk: all of a
sudden he wanted to take charge of our birth control
and use a condom. But after only a few weeks we
both agreed that neither of us liked it. I went back
to the diaphragm. Still, he checked to make sure that

I was wearing the contraption at every intercourse. It didn't matter how turned on he was: he always took just a moment to make sure I had it in. It was always in the back of his mind that I might just"forget" to use it, since I wanted a baby so badly.

There were times I didn't feel like having intercourse after "inspection." I never refused him, you understand, but sometimes the checking killed the mood.

As a matter of fact, the woman's occasional disinterest in engaging in intercourse has been clinically noted by Dr. Lidz of Yale. According to Lidz, what seems to be operating is frustration at having sexual intercourse "for no purpose" when contraception is used.[8]

Contraceptives don't always provoke such negative responses. Once women are confident they won't get pregnant (for example, when taking the Pill), many report increased zest for relations, a fact noted by many researchers.

For some, contraceptives provide benefits. One woman said that her husband's willingness to use condoms proved how much he loved and cared for her. He disliked using the prophylactic, but he didn't want to risk his wife's health by use of either the Pill or an IUD. A husband viewed his wife's use of a diaphragm—with the messiness and hassle it entailed for her—as a demonstration not only of her love for him but of her concern for their shared physical relationship, since it meant that *he* didn't have to use a condom.

Restoring equilibrium. Still, the most *equal* relationship is often found among couples using natural methods. There are reasons for this, of course.

At the beginning of this book, I pointed out that whenever artificial methods are used, a "shock" factor is involved; usually one partner must absorb most, if not all, of this shock. Certainly this is the case with oral contraceptives or the IUD. Only the woman's health—even her life—is at risk.

The only male birth control method that seems to pose a health hazard is a vasectomy.

Barrier methods, especially foam and diaphragm, are "messy"—something that troubles women considerably more often than men. All barrier methods are, of course, interruptive. Both partners must absorb the "shock" of such interruption to greater or lesser extents. But disequilibrium has been clinically noted: in one study, researchers found that some "coitus-connected methods"—condom and withdrawal—were discontinued because of objections by the husband. In contrast, there were no objections noted for either the diaphragm or for foam.

Natural methods have drawbacks—observing the fertility signs, charting them, coping with abstinence—but the difference is monumental: *these* drawbacks are shared.

6

How to Cope with Abstinence

Because it requires mutual coping, abstinence has turned into a bonus for all but a handful of couples. Indeed, the self-denial, discipline, and mutual sharing and decision-making have been a spur for both individual and mutual growth. A husband married fifteen years commented on this:

> In the beginning we thought that if my wife went on the Pill, the freedom of having intercourse as often as we wanted would bring us closer together. . . . But now that we are using NFP, our marriage is growing better every day. It didn't on the Pill. We've learned that there is more to marriage than sex.

Couple after couple have indicated that their relationships have become more intimate, have deepened. But very few expected such positive, apparently unrelated, rewards when they first set aside contraceptives, especially the couples who came to NFP classes out of desperation. One couple enrolled because the wife couldn't tolerate the Pill and had needed emergency major surgery for an IUD-related complication. The couple signed up for a course in natural family planning as a last resort. "When we learned how long the abstinence could be, it was a shock," the husband told me. "I said to my wife, 'Honey, we're never going to make it on this method.' After four months, I guess it's getting a little better, but it hasn't gotten easier. Maybe in another year or two I'll feel different."

Very likely the man will feel different in another year or two, according to Don and Sylvia Kramer, directors of the Twin Cities Natural Family Planning Center at North Memorial Medical Center in Minneapolis. The Kramers, too, came to NFP when there was nothing left. They had used calendar rhythm and all the major artificial methods—IUD, Pill, diaphragm—without any great degree of satisfaction. The only thing left was natural family planning.

Through their own experience the Kramers recognized that there are usually five stages in learning to cope with abstinence—the same five that Dr. Elisabeth Kubler-Ross identified for terminally ill patients dealing with their impending death. This may appear to be a bizarre comparison, but there are similarities: both are essentially *life struggle* situations. These five stages represent the normal human response to such situations, regardless of what form they take in our lives.

The five stages. Here's how the stages often unfold with respect to abstinence:

Stage 1—Denial. "Honey, we're never going to make it on this method" is the first stage. The feeling is that it *can't* be; that abstinence isn't *really* necessary, that there *must* be a way out. In other words, the reality is denied. When the couple accepts the fact that abstinence *is* part of natural family planning, they may then move into the second stage.

Stage 2—Anger. The couple may lash out at each other, fight, argue about other things, but their anger really stems from a feeling of being "conned" into use of a method that has such terrible restrictions. One or both partners may feel this anger in differing amounts. Generally, the anger disappears when the couple thinks they have found a way out; they've moved into stage 3.

Stage 3—Bargaining. The couple begins to accept the reality of the situation by trying to find ways to make it easier. "Okay, we've got to abstain. Let's see if we can shorten the days."

Sometimes the couple consults the chart together and discusses "taking chances." They may also decide to try using contraceptive barriers during the fertile time. This type of solution, however, makes the couple more acutely aware that intercourse is no longer completely natural. Something is "off," "not right," "missing." Couples previously on the Pill who enjoyed intercourse without any barriers find readjustment to artificial barrier methods too disheartening. And, of course, some couples using barrier methods during the fertile time are surprised by an unplanned pregnancy. So once a couple realizes there are no viable "bargains" they move into stage 4.

Stage 4—Depression. "Okay, we'll abstain. Abstinence never lasts *too* long, after all. There's always an end to it. It's really not that bad." Not exactly *empty* words, but hardly a cheering thought. And depression sets in. After all, it's hard—very hard—to be content with such an annoying situation. At this point, the couple is usually ready to move into the last stage.

Stage 5—Acceptance. It would seem that this stage is the best. But it's neither "best" nor "worst"; neither a happy stage nor an unhappy one. It just *is*. Both completely accept that they have a mutual responsibility and "job" to share with respect to family planning.

Dr. Viktor E. Frankl, internationally renowned psychiatrist, has pointed out in his new book, *The Unheard*

Cry for Meaning, that when we are no longer able to change *a situation,* we are challenged to change *ourselves.* If this challenge is accepted, the result is growth; we rise above ourselves, become more than we have ever been.[1] Indeed, this is what happens to the couple who accepts abstinence. *They can't change the situation, but they have the opportunity to act as partners in a growth process that inevitably accompanies the use of natural family planning methods, if the couple truly accepts the partnership.*

Of course, no one experiences these stages in exactly the same way. It takes months, sometimes years, for most couples to move from denial to acceptance. Some couples can move from denial to acceptance in one evening. Others skip several stages altogether; for example, they may start bargaining the first night they learn about natural family planning. There are also couples who are past bargaining; they're already too depressed.

Individual spouses aren't necessarily at the same stage at the same time. A husband can be angry and his wife depressed; a wife may be interested in bargaining while her husband has reached acceptance. The experience of the three following couples reflects the growth through the stages:

> We are in the process of writing a book which we hope will be helpful to other couples. In it we describe our personal struggle from viewing abstinence as a burden, to coping with it, to acceptance of it as being positive, to making it a creative part of our marriage, to becoming joyous about it! We have grown so much and to a great extent we believe that much of it has been because of NFP.

> When we first started using the method there was that longing for Phase III; now we are realizing a great happiness even during the abstinence. . . .

How super it is to run up to my husband and give him a big hug when he walks toward the house each evening. I feel like a young bride when I prepare one of his favorite meals and take walks in the new snow in the evenings followed by cuddling up in bed with a great feeling of being loved even though we are in a short time of abstinence. I always thought, "Well, life will begin when we reach the OK part of the cycle," but now I realize that life is special every day of the cycle.[2]

Our desire for intercourse is at its highest level during the most fertile days. It is nearly impossible for us to refrain on these days, but we are learning to manage. We used withdrawal—and I got pregnant with it once—but today we no longer use withdrawal at all.

The effects on our marriage have been good. Initially, my husband said that we would try NFP for six months and then we'd make a decision about whether or not to continue. NFP has forced us to communicate. This area has always been weak with us. We "grew up" so to speak by taking responsibility for our drives. The methods are highly satisfactory and I'd recommend them to other couples.

The Natural Birth Control Disequilibrium

It would be a pleasure to report that every couple passes more or less smoothly through the various stages, from denial, through anger, bargaining, and depression, to final acceptance. A pleasure to report—and far from the truth. For some couples, natural family planning can become a fresh battleground in the marital fray. A wife described what happened in her marriage:

My husband did not want to be "told when to have intercourse." So usually when I told him that it was safe, he would begin *his* period of abstinence. He was not going to be forced to make love by the calendar; he was not going to be used as my sex object.

This woman went on to write in her questionnaire that her husband didn't want to use condoms because they were too disruptive. "But I also refused to use a diaphragm because I felt it would be too disruptive," she added. "I feel about the diaphragm the way he feels about a condom." The woman also felt that the Pill and IUD were hazardous. Moreover, she was convinced that there was just something "right" about a natural method. "It makes sense to me that NFP allows one to be in touch with one's cycle, and without contraceptive barriers a couple is truly two-in-one."

But the husband's questionnaire revealed that he saw no advantage to natural methods; he thought that NFP was "unsafe" and that it killed spontaneity. He rated the method "unsatisfactory," would not recommend it to other couples, and felt that the effects had been negative.

It was a no-win situation: the wife had reached acceptance, but the husband remained angry. Despite the woman's misgivings and deepest wishes, the couple relied on a female-oriented barrier method during the fertile phase. As far as the wife was concerned, it was the only way to achieve a measure of peace in the marriage.

Dr. Max Levin, a neuro-psychiatrist and clinical professor at New York Medical College, commented at length about such situations in an issue of *Child and Family:*

When a man and wife are unhappily married, the smallest thing can loom up as a big problem. . . . In such a marriage periodic continence can become a major issue. The husband regards sex, not as something he can give his wife, but as something he can give *himself* as compensation for his various grievances.

In my own experiences there has been no exception; in the cases I have seen where periodic continence was presented as an intolerable burden, there has not been a single case where I didn't find something seriously wrong with the marriage. There was no love, no spirit of devotion. One or both partners were immature, egocentric, selfish. They were wrapped up in themselves, not in each other. It was not the frustration of the . . . method that was disturbing them [and they don't] need to use other contraceptive methods. They need therapy and counseling to find out what is wrong with their personalities and why the promise of their marriage has not been realized.[3]

Manipulation and control. Natural family planning can be used negatively: manipulation and control problems are not strangers to NFP couples. They are at the root of this wife's comments:

I guess my husband viewed me as the "victor" because we did not use contraceptives during four years in which we had two pregnancies. On the other hand, I felt he was the "victor" and a very effective fighter. We might not use contraceptives, but we had sex when HE was willing. Using NFP unilaterally really set me up: I was damned if I did and damned if I didn't. My husband took *no responsibility* in this area; any mistakes or pregnancies were my "fault" (to use his choice of words) .

It is not surprising that the woman's husband took no responsibility for the couple's family planning. It is symptomatic of severe disequilibrium that one partner—usually the wife—is left fielding the family planning responsibility alone.

Minor disequilibrium. Severe disequilibrium is usually symptomatic of other difficulties in the relationship. But even good relationships can be uneven in a different way:

> Long abstinence periods cause tension. During our short safe times I initiate sex oftener than I'd like because I know I'd better do it then before the long abstinence.

Another woman felt that her husband didn't trust her "calculations" yet, "possibly because I am so unsure of myself." This disturbance is likely to clear up with time, since the couple is new to NFP and is learning it in one of the most difficult circumstances: the lactation period after childbirth. As time goes on, perhaps the husband will become more involved in the "calculations"—to use the wife's word—and will become a true partner in the decision-making about fertility and infertility.

In another marriage, it was clear that the partners did not view fertility as a *shared* condition:

> Let me say first that there seems to be little resentments in marriage toward personalities or things said or done in the past. On top of that, I think that my husband holds me or my body responsible for his not being able to have sex. I feel frustrated not only at that responsibility but also for our not having sex. In addition, there are those *other* resentments underlying our talks or arguments when we're ostensibly talking about our frustrated sex problems.
> For example, he wants to play around during our unsafe periods more than I want to. Then *other*

problems or set-backs make him more aware of his sexual frustrations. As a result, we're sometimes having more than one argument in one fight—if that makes sense. In other words, we're ostensibly arguing about sex, but what's *really* causing the resentment is something that happened way back in our marriage.

Sometimes there's difficulty using natural family planning for the simplest, plainest, and most basic reason of all: abstinence is hard! One husband put it bluntly: "I'm too horny."

A letter from a young wife underscored the difficulty of abstinence:

> Although we will never go back to any other type of birth control, involvement with NFP is not a happily-ever-after story. It is sacrifice and a lot of self-control. After using the Pill, I'm still in the "mind-set" of if it feels good—do it. It's like going on a diet after pills used to keep me slim.
>
> And what do other women do with husbands that are pushy, don't trust the method, become angry at the wife for not being infertile, then are overly afraid of getting the wife pregnant? What about husbands who are generally frustrated because of lack of sex?
>
> We've got all the strains, and seemingly little of the enrichment, although there is some. If you catch us during the infertile time, we will possibly be more enthusiastic about NFP. Rationally, it does have everything else beat by a mile.

7

Why Abstinence Makes a Difference

It was a cliché of the early artificial birth control movement that if a couple could physically express their love at will, they would grow closer, strengthening their marriage. That promise seems not to have been realized. In contrast, many couples insist that it *has* been realized with a method that involves periodic abstinence. These comments are typical:

> I went through many kinds of pills, experiencing vomiting, migraines, irritation, dissatisfaction. I also felt used—an object used for sex. The memories of us and our marriage were not pleasant and when we went on NFP both we and our marriage improved. We tend to think our earlier problems were related to our birth control.

> The ever-present opportunity to have sex became a performance pressure that neither of us enjoyed. At the same time, we didn't feel close enough to talk about what was bothering each of us. We drifted apart. Our prayers became lonely ones—each of us had the attitude that God should help the other to change.

As a first step in exploring the value of abstinence, it's important to probe a sensitive area: why do we make love in the first place?

Why we make love. University of Michigan psychologist Dr. Judith M. Bardwick examined some of the reasons for love-making. In one study, women were asked specifically: "Why do you make love?"

Initial responses were more or less as expected. In other words, the women offered what they considered to be the "right" answers. But after some delicate probing, the researchers learned that all was not quite the way the women had first reported it.

Sex was rarely described as pleasurable in its own right. Instead, two responses were most common: first, sex was a way to demonstrate love in a relationship that the women hoped was mutual; second, if the woman withheld sex favors, the man would leave. "The fear of abandonment was the single most critical conscious fear," reports Dr. Bardwick.[1] Because this fear was so high, many women perceived a man's willingness just to hold her, without having intercourse, as a sign of love.

This theme was clear in most of my interviews. Many women specifically mentioned how much it meant to them that their husbands were willing to abstain for the sake of their mutual goals. This came out in the questionnaires too. "Strange as it may seem," one woman wrote, "the abstinence has had a positive effect on our marriage. I feel that my husband has to love me deeply in order to abstain." Another woman said: "I feel so secure and loved. My spouse loves me for *me* and not as a sex-bed partner. I know this because during our abstinence, he is still loving and faithful and has self-control."

Mutual commitment. This woman's comment touches on another fear noted by Dr. Bardwick: women fear that commitment to the relationship is not equal. Thus, for many women, a husband's willingness to abstain

is proof of his love and devotion. One young wife, aged
twenty-one, had a direct experience with her husband's
loving devotion:

> After my little girl's birth, I experienced a lot of
> break-through bleeding that made us abstain for
> weeks. During this period my husband and I sup-
> ported each other a lot. Without his understanding,
> determination, *love,* and will power, NFP would not
> have been part of our daily lives. We are very happy
> to be part of NFP.

But is the woman's husband equally happy "to be
part of NFP"? Apparently yes. The husband, aged twenty-
five, rated the method as "highly satisfactory" and noted
that "it has made us closer and has shifted the emphasis
of physical love to a more mature and rounded love for
each other."

Other husbands reported themselves pleased by the
mutuality, closeness, sharing, and equality that are an intrinsic part of the commitment to natural family planning:

> We've become much closer in our love because of
> this shared responsibility.

> Since using natural methods I feel more of the
> power and responsibility of sex, since both of us know
> exactly when to have or avoid sex to have or avoid
> children.

> Natural methods offer us a greater knowledge of our-
> selves and each other and make our fertility as a
> couple a joint responsibility.

Wives, too, are thrilled to have their husbands "on board" as committed equals in family planning:

> It's neat to feel that my husband is involved in birth control with me and it's not just me popping a Pill, or whatever.

> Both share. My husband does the charting, makes sure I've taken my temperature.

> I know my husband feels that NFP is highly satisfactory because he's so enthusiastic about it. He's always updating his knowledge, taking my temperature, charting and helping me to interpret. Sometimes the abstinence period gets me down, but my husband has the ability to really get me through it and into the infertile phase. *He* makes the method worthwhile.

Problem marriages. If abstinence is helpful for couples who have no marital difficulties, it can be a boon for those who do. Since most marriages have difficult periods, abstinence can be a sign of commitment that makes it easier for the couple to deal with real issues, real problems. A twenty-four-year-old wife married four years wrote:

> Abstinence seems to highlight certain problems in our marriage. But if we had not learned to use NFP, I believe that these problems would have been unidentified, remained under the surface, and would have ended up causing more difficulties.

Sexual disequilibrium. Some couples have problems bringing sexual drives and needs into sync. Often the wife is less interested in frequent relations. But interestingly, even when this is the case, acceptance of the "ban" can be fruitful for both partners, as one husband discovered:

> Before using NFP, I spent many evenings thinking about how I was going to convince Joyce to have intercourse that night. Meanwhile, she was thinking about how she was going to convince me that we *didn't* need it that night.
>
> Now that we're using NFP, many nights are spent discussing problem areas in our marriage—ourselves, the children, etc. Overall, I would never trade NFP for any artificial method because it has helped us together. I'm also relieved that my wife is not in any medical danger from side effects of the Pill.

A nineteen-year-old wife was also relieved from sexual pressures by the intercourse ban:

> We are both very open about the fact that I don't seem to want intercourse as much as he does, although I am definitely beginning to want it much more than I used to. This pleases both of us. The fact that I can't have it some of the time makes sex all the more enticing, but neither of us thinks that I'll ever be as horny as Lenny. We joke about how grateful I am that we used NFP because the abstinence lasts longer than a headache.

The woman's twenty-year-old husband said that he found abstinence somewhat difficult, "but if the alternative is the Pill or an IUD, we'll abstain." This couple had used condoms ("bargained" with the method) during the first two months of the marriage. However, there were serious reasons for avoiding pregnancy—he was still in school; they had no savings whatsoever—and two intercourses in which they (unintentionally) failed to use the condom frightened them. If they continued to "play around" with the method, they might have an unplanned pregnancy. The husband also felt that having played it "both ways"—without abstinence, then with it—that the "honeymoon" effect of renewing the physical relationship made for a more exciting, meaningful experience than "sex on demand." He acknowledged that abstinence is hard, but noted that "if it weren't difficult, having intercourse again wouldn't be so exciting either. It's hard to have it both ways."

Thus, for this young couple, the wife's need to have fewer acts of intercourse was equalized with the husband's need for more via the impartial intermediary of their choice of birth control. Neither spouse felt an imposition; the wife enjoyed a respite and her husband found the respite ultimately worthwhile.

Sexual dysfunction. While natural birth control can be helpful when there are no problems in the bedroom other than unequal desires, it is sometimes most helpful when there are problems of sexual dysfunction. Indeed, it has become a sex therapy cliché: the way to achieve a normal sexual act is to forbid it, while encouraging greater physical intimacy—touching, caressing, fondling—over a period of days or even weeks. Dysfunctions like primary and secondary impotence and premature ejaculation have been helped by the well-known technique of refraining from intercourse, though not from touching.

Implicitly, NFP encourages couples to explore nongenital, nonorgasmic means of expressing affection and love during the fertile phase. One wife said that this "mini-sex therapy" became the inadvertent "cure" for her husband's impotence:

> Things got so bad that I stayed on the Pill despite serious headaches. We felt that it was important that

if he could get and sustain an erection, there should be no need for an interruption that could ruin it. That canceled out any barrier methods.

Today we realize that our thinking placed Joe under an intolerable strain. He felt constantly pressured to produce an erection to please me, especially since I was having so many problems with the Pill.

But finally problems with the Pill became too great. If he managed an erection, I had a screaming migraine.

Matters have improved now that we can't have intercourse for almost two weeks. In fact, we almost didn't make it through the first abstinence phase, which astonished both of us. We bought condoms for the second one, but they created the old problem again: my husband felt the pressure to please me. Everything fizzled, pun intended.

Today we're not having as much intercourse as I would like, but I do enjoy the petting and touching. He does too. I also enjoy the fact that we're not always concentrating on *his* erection, *his* penetration, and whether or not *he* can keep going. Intercourse works out most of the time without our thinking about it—although we still have our flops.

I think that we both accept the reality of the situation, especially since things have improved over the past thirty-eight months that we've used NFP. My husband has become more accepting of his sexuality and his problems. I have too.

Another couple didn't wish to detail what their sexual problem (or problems) had been, but they found that fertility awareness helped them with the difficulty:

NFP has definitely been a help to certain physical problems in our marriage and has also helped our relationship. Sex used to be THE subject in our marriage and created a lot of pressure. Now it's back in a more supportive position. Also, when sex was THE subject, it wasn't very good. Now that it's more in the background, it's much, much better. It has freed us to be more comfortable with sex and each other. Now we're more open and talk about things more, especially since the performance pressure is off.

Sex is better. None of the couples I interviewed complained that abstinence had hurt the marriage. A few individuals made this complaint in the questionnaires, as noted in the previous chapter, but most reported that the short abstinence period renewed their zest. One young husband made an interesting comment when asked about drawbacks of NFP:

> The first and only "drawback" I can think of is the abstinence period. But after having used the method for twenty-two months, I can honestly say that the sexual tension created by the abstinence period is healthy and contributes to deeper sexual love between me and my spouse during the infertile phase.

A wife reported that abstinence restored romance:

> At certain times my husband tends to treat me more specially—like a fiancée rather than a wife. He doesn't take me quite so much for granted, like a cookie he can have anytime. I believe in some ways that abstinence keeps his mind from wandering to other women because he's anxious to have intercourse just with me. I respond to that by keeping up my appearance; I also make sure that my personality remains appealing to him.

It isn't just that abstinence whets the appetite. Others report that having learned fertility awareness, they feel more confident, relaxed, and responsive, since they're sure that conception can't occur. This is a reaction more common to women, although many men also reported it.

Extending foreplay. Many women derive much greater enjoyment from sexual relations when foreplay lasts longer. Men, too, find that extending foreplay can make the final orgasmic experience more explosive, more enjoyable. Thus, abstinence offers a double advantage for some: it builds excitement and tension *and* extends the foreplay, not only physically, but mentally. These comments are typical:

> My husband and I are much more affectionate and open, and we communicate better. Having intercourse isn't just something that happens at bedtime. We build up to it after a whole evening of togetherness.

> I used to think that I liked spontaneity. My wife and I have discovered that love-making is actually better when both plan and yearn for sex.

> Abstinence sharpens or rekindles my wife's attractiveness to me and prompts demonstrations of love and affection that I probably would neglect.

> We've both enjoyed the courtship during the time of abstinence and it's fun to prepare for the honeymoon when abstinence is over.

> I didn't like being Mrs. Availability the way I was with the Pill. There's a lot more mystery now with the abstinence. I like having the mystery—and believe it or not, so does my husband.

Dr. Donn Byrne points out that imagination is a vital element in sexual responsiveness.² Writing in *How Can a Man and Woman Be Friends?*, Mary Rosera Joyce points out that if the stimulus-response reflex is developed into a stimulus-*reflection*-response process, man's main sexual organ, the brain, becomes activated. When this happens, the human sexual experience has the potential to become greater, more all-encompassing. According to Joyce, "The spontaneity of sex is meant to be like the spontaneity of the fine arts, not like the impulsiveness of the child 'playing' the piano."³

The best insurance for this variety of spontaneity is *thought*. This bonus of the imaginative faculty is not as readily available to the couple that relies on contraceptives.

I received insight on this matter from one couple who tried to impose an abstinence period on themselves while they used the Pill. "The abstinence just got shorter and shorter and finally didn't exist at all," said the husband. "Sex became boring, and even though we both knew what was happening, we found that we just didn't have the motivation to abstain since we really didn't have to." Now that the couple are using natural family planning, they *do* have to abstain. And they have succeeded. "It makes all the difference," the husband admitted.

The Interpersonal Relationship

While many couples are surprised to find that their sexual relationship improves once they begin relying on natural family planning, an even bigger surprise may be what happens to their *interpersonal* relationship. There's a reason for this: once a couple mutually agree to use NFP, fertility awareness tends to uncover many matters that might have gone undiscussed, even undiscovered, by the spouses.

A wife described how the change to NFP helped to open better communications pathways:

> When we started using the methods, we really had to discuss a lot of new things. At first I wasn't sure how to interpret the changes in my mucus. We discussed that. Soon we were discussing how seriously we really wanted to forestall pregnancy. This came up especially during the times when abstinence was particularly difficult for one of us or both of us. In fact, we discussed the abstinence problem very extensively —how to cope creatively with the sexual tensions. We also planned how to enjoy intercourse after the abstinence period and our physical relationship took on a special excitement. We had never talked about things so intimately, so personally, or in such detail until we started using natural birth control.

The communication that develops can cover anything and everything: your sexuality, conflicts, goals, your marriage, your children, finances, other problems. Sometimes subtle things like attitudes and feelings that might otherwise have remained hidden emerge.

One couple made a discovery about sexual attitudes:

> The biggest surprise to me was the fact that *my wife* found the abstinence terribly difficult. I thought that I would have the problems—but I mean it: I practically had to tie her down to her side of the bed. She also became more aggressive as the abstinence came to an end and she let me know that she was looking forward to having intercourse again.
>
> I was terribly flattered to realize that my wife enjoyed relations with me so much. For years I had been grateful to her for always responding to my

"request" for intercourse. But after twenty-eight months of using natural methods, we finally see intercourse as something that we share and give to each other. She gives to me; I give to her.

It is important to discover that the wife is not the sole "giver of gifts." It's an awareness that places both partners on an equal footing.

Another couple made a different discovery about equality and responsibility in the first few years after they changed to fertility awareness methods:

> There were many times when I'd feel affectionate and loving and want to hug and kiss Jenny, or just give her a squeeze. But she'd freeze me out.
> Finally I said to her: "Okay, what's going on? What have I done? Why am I getting the big freeze?" You know what her answer was? That we were supposed to be abstaining; "Hey," I told her, "I'm in this too, you know. *I* know that we could get pregnant; I won't let anything get out of hand." Well, she knew that intellectually, but she still couldn't relax and trust me. Also, she didn't want us to get the least bit excited sexually because she worried about control—specifically *my* control. We worked out that problem for nearly three years. But now she trusts completely that I can—and will—handle our abstinence.

While this wife learned to trust her husband more within their marital relationship, she recognized that her earlier need to maintain their abstinence related to the fact that she had handled the couple's family planning for so long that she continued to feel responsible. In other words, the disequilibrium fostered by *her* prior use of the

Pill carried over when the couple changed to mutual family planning: she still felt solely responsible for insuring method effectiveness.

Growth adventure. Of course, many couples consider the abstinence quite enough "shared responsibility," but other couples go much further. In many cases the husband becomes intimately involved with the task of charting, even handling it completely. Indeed, one of the most impressive aspects of NFP involves the process of continual growth in the area of *mutual* responsibility—something that is quite distinct from individual responsibility.

One husband said that when he first heard about natural methods he was sure that they would be effective. Then he added: "However, I misunderstood my role. My wife had too much responsibility." The man's comment is indicative of a change from viewing family planning as "her" responsibility to viewing the responsibility as "ours."

The wife's questionnaire revealed more detail about this responsibility and the couple's growth:

> When we first started using NFP, my husband left everything up to me, including maintaining the abstinence, while sometimes trying to encourage me to "break the fast." I told him that I didn't mind "keeping the records" but that we both had to work at maintaining abstinence, and *not* by keeping at opposite ends of the house.
>
> It was after that, that we began to work at NFP together. I suppose this new closeness has been gradual, because I cannot tell you exactly when it began, but we are so much more open with each other and better able to communicate.

Total sharing. The mutuality involved in using fertility awareness can be so profound that it may subtly affect the thinking of a couple. It comes down to this:

men and women stop thinking of themselves as the "opposite" sex; they begin considering themselves the "complementary" sex. This change of thinking was revealed in a small but very important change in language—a fact I discovered accidentally during personal interviews. The subject of planning a pregnancy came up many times. I tended to direct this kind of discussion toward the woman—a reflection of my own culturally conditioned bias. But during one interview a husband told me about the couple's decision to use NFP to conceive and said: "The first time we tried it, it worked! We got pregnant."

We got pregnant. The phraseology jarred me. But a few interviews later, another husband mentioned that "we got pregnant." There it was again!

Having noted this phraseology crop up twice accidentally, I looked for it deliberately: when I could, I directed questions about the decision to conceive toward the husbands. Seventeen husbands used the plural form of that pronoun in connection with conception. That makes a total of nineteen husbands thinking in the plural about pregnancy, about 20 percent of the men interviewed.

What's more, I had already interviewed over a quarter of the couples before I noticed the two "we got pregnant" phrases used by husbands. As I already mentioned, because of my own bias, I had previously been directing all such questions to the women. I am convinced that if I had caught on sooner, I would have had a larger tally.

At heart, fertility awareness is a completely shared venture.

A Family Affair

The sharing that is involved in fertility awareness affects the entire family. Dr. Mary Ella Robertson, a sociologist who served on the Secretary's Advisory Committee on Population Affairs, U.S. Department of Health, Education, and Welfare, reports that the deeper bond of mutuality and commitment fostered between parents by their use of NFP ". . . not only dramatically improves the marital relationship, but [it] also makes it easier to rear the children. It is a subtle thing, but it's a very real thing: The children sense the commitment of the parents to each other and to them. It enhances the child's feeling that he or she belongs to a united family, one permeated by caring and love."

Other matters are uncovered. For example, the parental dialogue about sex is often made considerably easier. A mother told me her learning experience:

> My parents found it very hard to talk to me about sex. I found out everything from my cousins, not from my parents. But I'm not much different from my mother: I, too, find it difficult to talk to my children about sex. But the simple fact that we rely on NFP forces me and Bob to talk about sex and sexuality a great deal. I found that our discussions over the years have made me so comfortable with the subject that it has been easier than I would have ever expected for me to talk to my daughters about the changes in their bodies and what they mean. Even Bob has said that he feels surprisingly at ease when the girls ask him birds-and-the-bees questions. We both agree that this comfortable openness comes from the fact that we've grown to be completely uninhibited with each other about sex.

A mother found that NFP offered a realistic way to talk about pre-marital sex with her seventeen-year-old son:

> One night my youngest son was talking to me about his girlfriend. To my astonishment, he was actually

wondering out loud whether or not he should sleep with her. I don't know what surprised me more: that he was considering it—or that he was *telling* me that he was considering it.

But suddenly I knew just how I felt about premarital sex: I wanted my son's first sexual intercourse to take place under circumstances of mutual love and total commitment. That's how his father and I had had our first experience—on our wedding night.

I also realized why it had been so hard to deal with the subject with our oldest children. We had used the Pill, so it was fine for *us* to say, "Wait until you get married." The message was: "Don't have sex now; then after you get married, you can have all you want."

Now that we're using natural family planning the message is different: "You can't have intercourse anytime you please. Look at us: we're married and even *we* can't have intercourse whenever we want. And I know what you mean: sometimes it's very hard holding off. I can really sympathize with you because dad and I deal with the problem all the time."

What this mother discovered is that she and her husband are in equilibrium not only with each other but with their children. There were no "don't you dare!" harangues; instead, there was a communality, a feeling of "I know it's a problem for you because it sure is a problem for us."

A grade schooler's mother had a different experience:

Danny came home from fifth grade one day having received the school's mandatory sex lecture, complete with a full description of all the contraceptive paraphernalia that's available. I was *very* annoyed: I had wanted his sex education to come from us. Anyway, home he arrived, bright with this brand-new knowledge. Suddenly he asked me if I could tell him what daddy and I use for birth control.

It was the first time in my life that I was completely relieved that I wasn't on the Pill. I was able to tell my son that daddy and I don't use anything; that if we want to have intercourse during a time of the month that I could get pregnant, why, we just wait a week or two until I can't get pregnant anymore. Then when we *do* want to get pregnant, we wait for that time of the month when we're fertile.

Danny was very impressed by all of this. He told me that's the method he wants to use when he gets married, and that he'll wait until his wife is fertile when they want a baby. But when they have to postpone a pregnancy, they'll wait for the infertile time.

Already at age ten he's thinking in terms of mutual responsibility for sexual intercourse and family planning.

8

Artificial vs. Natural: How Do They Compare?

Some researchers worry that since natural methods do require the willingness to accept mutual responsibility, effectiveness will be reduced. What if there isn't an "equal" sense of responsibility?

This can be a problem—but it isn't unique to natural birth control: artificial methods are more effective when both man and woman are involved. As a matter of fact, family planning doctors and researchers are beginning to recognize that contraception is more effective when both spouses are interviewed. A joint interview makes the man aware that he, too, plays a role in the couple's birth control when it's artificial; even if it's just a passive role—as is usually the case—it's a *role*.

When men become involved, results are usually better, sometimes dramatically so. In a study in Iran, psychiatrist Iradj Siassi found that only 12 percent of 100 wives continued to take their oral contraceptives for six months when they were solely responsible. In contrast, an experimental group of 100 other couples showed a 93 percent compliance rate during the same six months. The difference? In the experimental group, *the husbands* were responsible for dispensing the Pill to their wives each day.[1]

While there may be a cultural element involved here, Dr. Judith Bardwick suggests a critically different dynamic: "If you want to predict the behavior and attitudes of women, then the best single variable is what they perceive are the attitudes and values of the men with whom they are involved. This would be the case even if they were professional and highly educated."[2]

Communication. Agreement to use natural methods does not insure their success. Another ingredient is required: good communication between the partners.

No birth control method, including artificial ones, is highly effective *unless* the couple can communicate. Two researchers have correlated contraceptive success rates with high communication skills.

Dr. Cornelius B. Bakker and Cameron R. Dightman have found that marital discord can lead to "forgetting" to take the Pill. "Forgetting" also relates to conflicting attitudes toward sexuality—another symptom of inability to communicate and resolve conflict.[3] For example, a wife may feel "used" during the sex act, particularly if her husband refuses to engage in foreplay or makes only perfunctory attempts. Rather than bringing her needs and desires into the open, she may decide to "get something" out of the act of intercourse—in this case, a baby—by "forgetting" to take her Pill.

Unplanned pregnancies are also linked to an inability to create or maintain a satisfying interpersonal relationship. Researchers have noted reasons for this—an echo of Dr. Bardwick's observations about abandonment fears: ". . . Such an inability may make a woman more dependent upon intercourse as a compensatory strategy for maintaining closeness, or deficiencies in communications skills may make it impossible to discuss clearly and responsibly the issues of contraception."[4]

Maturity. Researchers point out that natural birth control methods have a drawback: they require maturity and stability on the part of both spouses. This is true; this is also true of effective users of contraceptives.

Dr. Peter Barglow, a psychiatrist with Chicago's Northwestern University Medical School, has found that women practice contraception much more effectively if they are mature—a finding ratified by Dr. Cornelius B. Bakker and Cameron R. Dightman. "Immature women who have a tendency toward acting out and who avoid taking responsibilities are prone to forget their contraceptives," they report.[5] Even the ability to tolerate oral contraceptives seems to be related to psychosexual maturity.

One reason teen-age unwed pregnancy rates are so high is that the partners are not only manifestly immature, but are also unable to perceive reality accurately. The it-can't-happen-to-me syndrome is rampant and reflects an unrealistic evaluation of action and consequences consistent with an immature, even childish, world view.

Impulse gratification—an important measurement of immaturity—is higher in women who have higher rates of unplanned pregnancies. Women who have a capacity to postpone gratification, to delay the satisfaction of impulses, are better candidates for using natural methods. Paradoxically, this capacity is also necessary for women to practice contraception effectively. Artificial birth control may make it possible to satisfy sexual urges immediately, but ironically, the woman who doesn't have the capacity to defer sexual pleasure is not a good candidate for effective contraception!

While maturity, good communication skills, and willingness to share responsibility are necessary for effective use of contraceptives, it should be noted that individuals with certain kinds of disturbances also use artificial birth control effectively. For example, a woman with an abnormal fear of pregnancy won't "forget" her contraceptives. Neither will certain kinds of anxious individuals. Extremely dependent women are effective users of artificial methods if their partners want them to be. And the obsessive-compulsive personality type is an ideal candidate for effective contraception.

Other drawbacks. It has been suggested that natural family planning methods are successful only for couples in committed, *married* relationships. One of the questionnaire respondents made a comment about this:

> I introduced this method to a single friend who leads a fairly active sexual life. She felt that it was a good method for someone who has a steady partner (such as a spouse) because a permanent relationship then exists and the period of abstinence can be dealt with. For someone without such a partner, she felt that NFP would not be a choice method, because the "current partner" may not understand or trust the method and may want to deal with the fertile period by using some artificial method.

Even the Department of Health, Education, and Welfare has listed the commitment aspect of NFP as one of its disadvantages. Notes HEW: "Women who are not committed to a long-term sexual relationship may not be able to have cooperation of a male partner."

Yet Dr. Peter Barglow, among others, has pointed out that married people tend to use artificial birth control more successfully than unmarried people. One reason for this, according to Dr. Barglow, is that the ability to maintain a prolonged relationship produces a relatively low number of partners. Consequently, the number of exposures to new situations—when one may or may not be prepared with contraceptives—is diminished. "This is consistent with proper planning for the bearing of children. It also correlates with the capacity to do something skillfully over a long period of time," Barglow reports.[6] Other researchers point out again and again that unmarried people—and not just teen-agers—are poor users of contraceptives.

The role of commitment. The fact that fertility awareness methods can only "work" in a relationship with some commitment may explain why I met so few single people relying on natural birth control. Three singles spoke to me about their use of the methods: one man and two women. In none of the cases did I speak to or meet the respective partners. In contrast to the married couples, none of the three even suggested that I get in touch with the partner.

NFP teachers tell me that occasionally single people come into the classes, but not often as couples. Usually the woman comes unaccompanied; her motivation, to discontinue the Pill.

When an unmarried couple attends classes together and practices NFP, their relationship often undergoes a change very quickly: either they break up, or they become more committed, often marrying.

Becoming more committed, even marrying, is not only related to the growing closeness these methods foster; facing abstinence *together* also helps each partner see the other as a unique, very special individual. And as Dr. Viktor E. Frankl points out, "Grasping the uniqueness of a loved one understandably results in a monogamous partnership. The partner is no longer interchangeable."[7]

There is another element involved—a critical one illuminating the vast difference between artificial and natural birth control. According to Dr. George E. Maloof, a psychiatrist affiliated with the North San Mateo County Mental Health Center in the San Francisco area, artificial methods "may lock a couple into an arrested state of marital development wherein their feelings are not shared." In such a case, the couple's interpersonal problems simply are not confronted. In contrast, natural family planning methods not only enable the couple to share and communicate, *but the methods themselves can actually serve as an aid to that sharing and communication if the couple mutually agree to use them.*

In other words, if you have difficulties talking, sharing, and communicating your feelings, your ambivalence about pregnancy, conflicts about your sexuality, as well as other problems related to your intimate relationship, you may find that the use of natural methods will help you open up, and do so *at a rate that can be comfortably accommodated by each of you.*

Deepening marital joy. Of course, natural family planning is not solely for couples who have interpersonal difficulties. Indeed, couples who already have a good relationship are usually surprised by how much better it becomes. "We were always a close couple," said a woman married eleven years. "But I can't believe how much closer we've become in the last three years since we started relying on fertility awareness. In fact, my husband told me that he feels we've grown more intimate during the past forty months than during all the previous years of our marriage put together. I agree."

For another couple, the decision to share the responsibility—and cope with the abstinence—brought the spouses closer, deepening their communication:

> My husband was anxious to try anything besides what we were using. He was also ready to make birth control a mutual responsibility.
>
> Despite the fact that I have difficulty abstaining when I'm ovulating, the advantages far outweigh this one hurdle. Perry is aware of this and is very understanding, trying to be more affectionate in other ways. However, we are growing the longer we use the method.
>
> I have to realize that he is trying not to become

"turned on" at the wrong time and might even act aloof, forgetting that I need more affection, not less, during abstinence. This is a struggle for us, but one in which we've both become more aware of each other and our feelings and attitudes about sex. We have become closer through the communication we've had to have in order to be successful with this method.

Another wife's reaction was summed up in a single sentence—"I now know the true meaning of the word 'intimate.' "

The heart of the matter. Intimacy is the most important goal of all our deeply held romantic aspirations. Our vulnerability lies in the fact that true intimacy cannot be achieved alone; rather, it depends completely, totally, 100 percent on *another*. Since acceptance of abstinence within the marital bed implies love, trust, and confidence in each other and in a shared future, this may be one reason why many men, and especially women, "blossom" emotionally and sexually after the couple begins to rely on fertility awareness. As the world-famous psychologist and father of self-actualization, Dr. Abraham H. Maslow, has pointed out, "The people who can't love don't get the same kind of thrill out of sex as the people who can love."[8]

There is evidence for Maslow's view in a recent study published in the *New England Journal of Medicine*. Of 100 couples described as predominantly happily married, researchers noted that any sexual "difficulties" experienced by the couples "probably reflected interpersonal problems to which both the husband and the wife contributed." The researchers also found that sexual dysfunctions reflected various problems, educational "deficits," conflict within the relationship, inhibitions, and physiological difficulties. They concluded that "it is not the quality of sexual performance but the affective tone of the marriage that determines how most couples perceive the quality of their sexual relations."[9]

The same phenomenon was noted nearly two decades ago by researcher Lee Rainwater. In one study Rainwater found that when there is mutuality in the genital relationship, it is usually accompanied by a deeper satisfaction and security within the marriage.[10]

Do couples using natural family planning methods achieve deeper satisfaction and marital security? Judging from what the couples *say*, it would appear to be the case; judging from what they *do*, the evidence may be overwhelming.

One statistic will summarize what I mean.

One hundred and fifty-seven men and women returned questionnaires. These individuals were a diverse group geographically and had widely different educational, social, and religious backgrounds. (Several respondents specifically pointed out that they were not Catholic, lest I suspect a religious basis for their positive response to NFP.) The couples had only one thing in common: they had learned to use natural family planning methods during or, in the case of a handful of the newly married couples, prior to marriage.

The divorce rate for this sampling of married couples was 0.6 percent. In other words, *less than 1 percent of the respondents had been previously married and divorced!* Specifically, only one individual out of 157 who responded had been divorced.*

This was a first marriage for 154 respondents; two respondents had been previously widowed.

Why such a low divorce rate? What makes the difference? It's difficult to say. One thought that came to mind

---

* Seven additional questionnaires were received after this section was written. No previous divorces were reported in those seven.

was that a large percentage of the couples were Catholic. The Roman Catholic Church remains the only major Western religious body that forbids divorce and remarriage. But even if all the respondents were Catholic—which they weren't—the explanation is weak. Writing in the June, 1978, issue of *U.S. Catholic,* Monsignor Steven J. Kelleher reports: "There are at least six million divorced Catholics in the United States; almost half of them have remarried. The proportion of divorces among Catholics is approximately the same as that among Jews and Protestants: from one-third to one-half of all marriages."

Another explanation for the low divorce rate is the possibility that the marriages were only a few years old. One expects that most couples can tough it out for at least a *few* years.

Unfortunately, not even that answer will wash: only 30 percent of the couples had been married six years or less; 40 percent had been married between six and eleven years; 30 percent had been married eleven years or more. *Thus, 70 percent of the couples represented had been married six years or longer.*

Several users of natural family planning suggest that the growing divorce rate is somehow related to widespread use of contraceptives. The questionnaire datum would seem to support this thesis but for one problem: the majority of the respondents had used artificial birth control at one time in their marriage. Moreover, some kind of self-selection is involved in changing to NFP. A couple with a deeply troubled marriage who are completely unable to communicate are not likely candidates even for learning, much less using, natural family planning.

Still, this datum reveals . . . something. One thing is certain: use of natural family planning is not harmful to a couple's relationship. But other questions are less certain: can natural family planning improve marriages? Increase marital and family happiness? Could it be a significant factor contributing to the permanence of a marriage? While the answers to those questions are less certain, I remember something said by James B. McDaniel, Jr., M.D., a staff member of the Buffalo Planned Parenthood Center in Buffalo, New York. Speaking of a method that involves periodic abstinence, Dr. McDaniel said: ". . . it is based on some of the finest qualities in man, namely, self-restraint, discipline, and responsibility."

Indeed, the qualities required to build a lasting marriage.

9
Looking to the Future

Natural family planning providers are beginning to recognize that they are dealing with considerably more than a birth control method. This is because the primary focus of natural methods is the couple—not a device. For NFP to be effective, both the man and the woman must agree to use the method and thereafter they must become—and remain—cooperative partners.

NFP is also uncovering new dimensions in the male-female sexual relationship. One of these is that a short abstinence phase seems to enhance, not detract from, the relationship. Dr. David E. Landers of Teaneck, New Jersey, an obstetrician and gynecologist with a deep interest in natural family planning, offers one explanation for this enhancement factor.

According to Dr. Landers, the primitive biological urge, human sexual energy, can be "harnessed" by us. Once harnessed, it can then be used to express whatever we want it to express, ideally love, joy, tenderness, empathy . . . all the positive human emotions.

Abstinence actively helps harness this energy. Like any energy source, sexual energy is more effective if "stored," to be released later at an appropriate time of our choice.

Sexual energy release is most readily triggered by the erotic. But that is also the most superficial "trigger." According to Dr. Landers, periodic abstinence helps the couple grow so that ultimately the "triggers" releasing sexual energy become the emotional and affective aspects of the couple's love bond. As a result, the erotic gradually loses its position as the primary sexual force. Instead, the *other person,* the loved one, plus the emotions and feelings felt toward the loved one becomes the primary force. Thus, the couple's life *together*—their joys, shared difficulties, achievements and milestones, headaches and heartaches—these life experiences can become the "power centers" of the sexual relationship.

Eventually, "person-centered" sexuality becomes a new sexual behavior pattern. But unlike the primitive sexual urge, it is *not* an instinctive behavior pattern: it must be learned. Moreover, the learning depends on sexual energy control.

Certainly one reason so many have become enthusiastic about NFP is that they have begun to master the art of sexual energy control. One woman commented on the positive effects on her marriage:

> When we *can* make love, my husband is more affectionate and tender and gentle. He is affectionate every day and looks forward to when we can make love. I don't feel "used" anymore and know he doesn't take advantage of sex *or* me.

Dr. James Fox, also a gynecologist-obstetrician practicing in Teaneck, New Jersey, points out other aspects of natural family planning. According to Dr. Fox, NFP is a method that operates simultaneously on at least three levels: the technological, the physical, and the interpersonal.

The technological level. Like contraception, natural

family planning is highly reliable when used properly. Unplanned pregnancies are rare, and at the same time, the method has no known hazardous side effects. In other words, from the point of view of sheer "technology" the method *works,* it's effective.

The physical level. I never interviewed an individual or a couple who complained that their sexual relationship had deteriorated because of their acceptance of abstinence. This complaint did appear twice in the questionnaires, but couples overwhelmingly report that their physical relationship had improved, sometimes considerably, since relying on NFP.

Certainly one reason for improvement is that the couples are "storing" their sexual energies. As one woman married less than a year said, "Abstinence is the best aphrodisiac." Obviously contraception doesn't involve any kind of storage and may be a factor in the growing problem of sexual boredom and male impotence.

Another matter: women often felt "used" while using contraceptives, particularly since many husbands tended to forget about "courting" them. Once they learned that their husbands were willing to abstain for a short period of time—in effect, not "use" them; rather, court them— their response became more ardent when intercourse became available again.

The interpersonal level. The human sexual experience is never wholly separated from the personal experience. Moreover, there are many ways to use sexual intercourse. It can be used for exploitation, conquest, humiliation, anger, etc. But ideally, sexual intercourse should be an expression of the deeper human emotions. Love, joy, spiritual closeness, tenderness, and other deep emotions that move men and women are profoundly suitable for sexual expression, although this is by no means the exclusive, or even the best, mode of expression. A touch, a glance, a soft smile, may say considerably more.

Most couples understand this instinctively, even though our culture tends to obscure this reality. Still, this instinctive understanding may be one reason why couples are willing to walk into an NFP class: couples already know that abstinence will be involved, but their values are sufficiently developed that "sex on demand" is no longer an essential value to them. It may still be *important* —and a cause of early difficulties with natural family planning—but it's no longer an *essential* value.

A young husband's experience shows how he and his wife began to experience natural family planning at all its levels:

> I never thought that after ten years of marriage and a handful of children I would ever feel the yearning for my wife that I had felt when we courted and were first married. I figured that all those old feelings were a part of being young and in love. Being older and loving each other was nice, but there certainly wasn't any cha-cha-cha about it.
>
> I wasn't enthusiastic when we changed to NFP, but we saw no other way. We went to class very, very reluctantly. Me especially.
>
> But almost right away it started happening again: that incredible yearning I used to feel for my wife returned—and not just once in a while: it was there every month. Every cycle gradually turned into courtship and honeymoon all over again.
>
> We think that the longing and yearning we feel for each other is better than what we felt when we were younger. We both think this is because we've been through so much together by now—childbirth, baby's first steps, family weddings, as well as unemployment, sickness, and other hard times. NFP has become more than a method of birth control for us: it's a life style.

A woman was ebullient in summarizing her experience of NFP in the couple's life:

Our marriage "began" and bloomed 100 percent after we started using NFP. We felt closer to God and this helped our marriage. We had the phases of courtship and honeymoon and celebrated. We shared my body awareness. We shared days of uncertainty and we shared days of gambling and pregnancy. It was a change from "I" to "we." Our last baby was conceived out of love, and with full knowledge that we would conceive. From that moment we could picture the hours and days of growth.

But before NFP I *feared* going to bed, as I didn't know my fertility cycle and worried that I might become pregnant. Now I know my fertility signs and feel 100 percent confident in those signs and no longer fear. It is a great relief and a burden off my shoulders. I want more children—but when I am ready and capable.

I would like to make a personal comment at this time. When I first heard about natural family planning, I thought of it as a last resort for couples who simply could not tolerate (for reasons of health) the effective artificial methods. And except for those with moral objections to contraception, it was unimaginable to me that any couple would actually *prefer* a natural method to an artificial one.

Today I recognize that periodic abstinence is not only effective for fertility control, it is also a creative contribution to the human experience. Personally, I can no longer imagine any other love style but this one. It is my hope that this, too, will become your discovery.

II

How to Start Charting Tomorrow

10

Keeping Your Charts

There is one urgent recommendation to make at the outset: seek competent, *personal* instruction. While I have met many couples who have learned to practice natural family planning from how-to books, personal guidance is always preferable. Appendix A lists referral addresses of teaching couples and centers throughout the United States and Canada.

If you seek personal instruction, you may have to select between two different approaches. The Ovulation Method (sometimes known as the Mucus-only or Billings Method) relies exclusively on the observation of the changing quality of cervical mucus. The Sympto-Thermal Method combines all the fertility signs. This book, of course, offers a Sympto-Thermal approach.

I selected this approach because studies comparing the two methodologies have consistently shown higher use-effectiveness rates for various formulations of the Sympto-Thermal Method. Ovulation Method use-effectiveness figures are generally lower—sometimes considerably lower—when calculated according to standard statistical practice. The discrepancy is currently under exploration inasmuch as the biological- or theoretical-effectiveness rates seem to be about the same for most formulations of both methods.

At any rate, if you obtain personal instruction, your teachers may give you slightly different guidelines or express the same ones differently. If this is the case, *follow the guidelines of your teachers.* The teaching of natural family planning is undergoing constant improvement. With competent, well-informed instruction, you will be the beneficiary of the latest research information available.

If there is no way for you to get personal instruction, *follow this book carefully.* It has been designed to be completely self-instructional. Both partners, the wife *and* the husband, should read all of Part I and the relevant portions of Part II.

As for charting, it takes far less time than inserting a diaphragm and at the same time offers potential for communication. For one couple, it's a positive experience they deliberately take time to enjoy:

> We've tried to keep up a daily dialogue. Our charting
> allows us a very special five to ten minutes during
> the day to discuss our personal and sexual feelings
> and their causes. We've always been an open, loving,
> touching couple—but stress of everyday life can
> hinder this. Charting helps us to grow!

It is up to the couple to decide how they wish to handle the charting, of course, but my recommendation is that the husband take charge of it. Personal and sexual communication is usually better when men handle this responsibility. So is charting. As one wife told me: "He asks, 'Do you mean somewhat translucent or actually clear mucus?' I'm forced to define the mucus change more precisely. The fact that my husband is 'on the team' really helps." One husband took such complete responsibility that his wife's gynecologist had to telephone him during a routine examination to find out when her next menstrual period was due!

Once you learn how to chart signs and recognize the fertile and infertile phases, you will be able to sever yourselves completely from the doctor and/or the drugstore in handling your family planning. Above all, natural family planning is *personal* control.*

Getting Started

You can begin your practice of natural family planning at this moment. In doing so, there is only one "rule" to keep in mind: *If in doubt—you're fertile.*

If you follow this important rule, you will never have to worry about an error in determining your fertility or infertility. This is because you must consider yourselves fertile *until you can prove you are infertile.* Thus, *at this moment,* you must "consider" yourselves fertile.

If you wish to avoid pregnancy, not even a drop of semen can come in contact with the female external genitals. (See page 40.) This requirement rules out not only sexual intercourse but all genital-genital contact until the couple can prove infertility.

What constitutes proof of infertility? When can you stop considering yourselves fertile? When you're beginning, the only positive proof of infertility is a *sustained basal body temperature rise* according to a specific formula —the rule of "6 and 4 and 3." (This rule will be explained below.)

Some women experience so-called "intermenstrual bleeding" episodes. These bleeding episodes do NOT follow ovulation. Indeed, it is possible for a woman to ovulate—and thus conceive—during such a bleeding. *So*

---

* The personal control aspect of NFP is discussed at length by author Mary Shivanandan in *Natural Sex* (Rawson, Wade Publishers, Inc.). See her chapter "The Medical Profession and Natural Methods."

UNLESS the couple is checking temperature to confirm the return of infertility, any bleeding experienced by the woman must always be considered fertile. Only a previous sustained temperature rise can prove otherwise. You will be using the "6 and 4 and 3" formula during your first learning cycle. Later, you will learn to chart the cervical mucus changes, evaluating two indicators according to the guidelines Dr. Roetzer has devised. With two fertility signs to cross-check, it will be possible to determine infertility earlier in most—but not all—charts.

But before moving ahead, it's essential to get a good foundation in temperature taking. Here's the important background information you require:

Taking your temperature. Your *waking* temperature is really what is meant by the term "basal body temperature." You should have at least three hours of sleep before taking it, and it should be taken immediately when you wake. Don't get up and do anything—including going to the bathroom—until after you've taken your waking temperature.

Your thermometer. Don't use a regular fever thermometer. Buy a BBT (basal body temperature) thermometer at your local drugstore—they cost about five or six dollars. A BBT thermometer is much more accurate, and the numbers are bigger and easier to read.* Don't use a BBT thermometer if you suspect you have a fever (more about fevers in the following chapter) and never wash it in anything but *cool* water.

How to take your temperature. You can take your temperature orally, rectally, or vaginally. You must, how-

---

* If you would like to cut temperature-taking time to approximately *thirty seconds,* you may wish to purchase the battery-powered Kenkoh electronic thermometer. Order for sixty dollars post-paid from The Human Life Center, St. John's University, Collegeville, Minn. 56321. (Minnesota residents add 4 percent sales tax.)

ever, be consistent in each cycle. Thus, if you start with oral readings at the beginning of your cycle, don't switch to vaginal or rectal readings later in the same cycle. Generally, these readings are a bit higher than the oral ones. You still get the same rising *pattern,* of course, no matter which orifice you use. Just use the same one in each cycle.

How to take oral temperatures. Oral temperatures should be taken for a full eight to ten minutes to insure an accurate reading on your BBT thermometer. Don't smoke or drink before taking your temperature. If you do drink something, *its* temperature may affect the temperature in your mouth and thus distort the readings.

On the other hand, if you happen to wake up an hour early, drink a glass of water, and return to bed, the temperature won't be distorted when you wake up again. Enough time will have elapsed so that the thermometer can reflect a proper waking temperature provided you take your temperature for the full ten minutes.

How to take vaginal and rectal temperatures. Lie in bed to take either vaginal or rectal temperatures. For rectal especially, lie in an S-shape on your side.

Sometimes you may need Vaseline or some other lubricant to slide the thermometer into the rectum. Use whatever seems to work best.

Rectal and vaginal temperatures need be taken for only five minutes to insure accurate readings.

Temperature taking and napping. Many women like to nap for the five minutes of temperature taking—eight to ten minutes if you're taking it orally. I urge you to stay awake, especially if you are relying on oral temperatures. You do *not* want your thermometer to break.

If you should happen to fall asleep, you may wind up taking your temperature for a much longer period than usual. This won't affect the reading, according to Dr. Edward F. Keefe, developer of the Ovulindex thermometer. However, the risk of breakage remains.

Is there a solution? One couple came up with an idea that seems to cut the risk of possible breakage, since the snooze—and the rectal temperature taking—is cut off precisely after five minutes. They keep an ordinary kitchen timer next to their bed. It's set for the five minutes of temperature taking and the ringing of the timer reawakens them. This couple follows the same routine on mornings when they sleep late. The temperature is taken at the usual time. The thermometer is removed five minutes later when the timer rings; the couple goes back to sleep for the rest of the morning.

Keeping a record. After you've taken your temperature, the reading must be recorded on a chart. (Free charts are included when you buy an Ovulinnex thermometer.)

Many husbands who handle the charting take care of it at night. If you choose to do it that way, be sure of one thing: set the thermometer aside somewhere where *it won't be exposed to heat.* It should be kept away from a radio, electric light or clock, radiator, etc.

After the temperature has been recorded, always shake down the thermometer. Grasp it near the end where the numbers are highest, hold tight, and give four or five good shakes to make sure that the mercury slides back down toward the bulb.

It is best to shake down the thermometer the preceding night so that it will be ready for you in the morning.

What readings to expect. This book will rely on Fahrenheit (F.) temperature measurements rather than centigrade (C.). Most women have a waking oral temperature of about 97.3° or so before ovulation. But don't be surprised if your waking temperature is as low as 96.7° or as high as 97.7°. (And remember: rectal and vaginal temperatures are generally higher than oral, sometimes as much as a degree.)

It's best to take your temperature at the same time each morning. If you do take your temperature forty-five minutes to an hour later than usual, make a notation on your chart. Usually the reading is about 0.1° higher for each hour later.

You can also expect higher-than-normal-temperatures if any of the following conditions prevail: you

- Slept restlessly;
- Were wakened several times during the night ("restless night");
- Had several alcoholic drinks the night before (and usually don't);
- Are taking special medication, especially hormonal-type medication);
- Are under severe emotional stress;
- Are ill;
- Used an electric blanket.

Such situations are known as "disturbances." I'll explain what you should do about them after discussing the application of the "6 and 4 and 3" guideline in the following pages.

As mentioned earlier, you are fertile until you can prove otherwise. For your first learning cycle, the only reliable proof that fertility has passed is the sustained temperature rise according to the "6 and 4 and 3" guideline.

Here's how to apply the guideline:

You are infertile on the evening you have recorded three *consecutive* waking temperatures all of which are at least 0.4° above the highest of the six lowest *consecutive* waking temperatures recorded before the rise began.

Thus, you are "looking" for two sets of temperatures: one low set and one high set. The low set must precede the high set, of course, and *all three temperatures* in the high set *must be at least 0.4° higher than the highest of the six temperatures in the low set.*

It is only when the above requirements have been met that you can reliably consider yourselves to be infertile. You *cannot* consider yourselves infertile before that. Only the sustained temperature rise according to the "6 and 4 and 3" guideline can be considered to be "proof" of infertility in your first charting experience.

Mucus changes. While you're waiting for the temperature rise, check for developing mucus. Some women, of course, worry that they won't be able to notice the changes. Of all the stories I've heard about learning to recognize mucus, Sheila Kippley offered the best expression:

. . . I have come to think that most women have not thoroughly learned the mucus observation until they become "aware" of its presence chiefly by external sensation. Seeing mucus on toilet paper is an additional aid but it is frequently not necessary in the overall picture of "becoming aware."

By "becoming aware," I mean a woman learns that mucus is present as she wipes herself; without looking she feels upon wiping that the external surfaces of the vagina are wet and slippery. Or she suddenly feels wet while shopping, gardening or doing other ordinary day-to-day activities. We can compare our "becoming aware" to other observations. One who brushes her teeth after eating or has an apple or carrot develops a feeling for clean teeth. It bothers her to have sweets without any follow-up dental care as she has learned to dislike the feeling of "dirty" teeth. Again, a person easily becomes aware of the feeling of dry, clean skin as opposed to sweaty, sticky skin. A person who cooks "feels" the difference between water and oil and doesn't have to see them to note a difference.

When I was first learning mucus awareness, I felt I didn't have any mucus externally and that an internal exam was necessary to find anything at all. I didn't feel I could learn to rely upon the sensation of vaginal wetness or lubrication. I found later, however, that to learn this sensation it must be *thought about constantly* throughout the day *at first.* The best and easiest way to do this is for a woman to try to sense what she can feel when wiping herself because this is something every woman does now and then during the day. After a few months of this, she can make this observation almost automatically and without thinking. The observation is now well learned, and she has developed a simple body awareness of her fertility. As one who went from "no mucus" to 7 to 9 days of mucus prior to ovulation, I feel many other women—*with effort at first*—can also learn to sense their mucus on the days before ovulation.[1]

Check for developing mucus each time you go to the bathroom. Wipe yourself before urinating to see if you get the slip-through feeling or can actually see mucus. Become alert to the changes, but don't worry about recording them during this first cycle. Just get used to noticing them.

Caveats. If you're on the Pill, mucus observations are worthless, since the hormones in oral contraceptives may act on the cervical mucus. If you are using an IUD and having problems with it, there may be a discharge that will conflict with the mucus signs. Thus, *you should not* *attempt to learn mucus changes if you are still relying on either one of these artificial methods.*

A couple observing mucus changes to determine fertility and infertility should never use foam or a diaphragm (with accompanying cream or jelly). These products may lead to confused interpretation of the cervical mucus changes.

Treated condoms have other difficulties. Some women have allergic reactions to the chemicals. Even untreated condoms can cause problems; some women have allergic reactions to the prophylactic itself.

Never use deodorant tampons. The chemicals used in the deodorant sometimes create problems (irritation, allergic reactions, etc.) that may obscure the mucus sign. Vaginal deodorants should also be avoided for the same reason. In actual fact, a healthy vagina is "self-cleaning" and should not emit an offensive odor, assuming normal, proper bathing of the vulva. If you notice an unpleasant odor, it may be an indication of pathology and should be checked by a doctor, *not* "treated" with a deodorant.

Antibiotics and antihistamines may also change the cervical mucus. If you are using any of these drugs, exercise extra awareness.

Chart No. 1. On page 125, you will find the complete waking temperature record for a woman with a thirty-four-day cycle. (Note: the calendar *dates* are entered in the left-hand column; cycle *days* are entered in the right-hand column.) Use this chart to test your understanding of the "6 and 4 and 3" guideline, and work out which day the couple could prove infertility.

Don't get flustered by all the temperatures on the chart; break the task into three easy steps:

First.   Look for the six lowest *consecutive* temperatures (the "low set") and draw a line

Chart No. 1*

A typical temperature chart

Date	Readings and Notes	
mar 3	9 97 1 2 3 4 5 6 7 8 9 98 1 2 3 4 5 6 7 8 9 99 1	1
4	9 97 1 2 3 4 5 6 7 8 9 98 1 2 3 4 5 6 7 8 9 99 1	2
5	9 97 1 2 3 4 5 6 7 8 9 98 1 2 3 4 5 6 7 8 9 99 1	3
6	9 97 1 2 3 4 5 6 7 8 9 98 1 2 3 4 5 6 7 8 9 99 1	4
7	9 97 1 2 3 4 5 6 7 8 9 98 1 2 3 4 5 6 7 8 9 99 1	5
8	9 97 1 2 3 4 5 7 8 9 98 1 2 3 4 5 6 7 8 9 99 1	6
9	9 97 1 2 3 4 5 6 7 8 9 98 1 2 3 4 5 6 7 8 9 99 1	7
10	9 97 1 2 3 4 5 6 7 8 9 98 1 2 3 4 5 6 7 8 9 99 1	8
11	9 97 1 2 3 4 5 6 7 8 9 98 1 2 3 4 5 6 7 8 9 99 1	9
12	9 97 1 2 3 4 5 6 7 8 9 98 1 2 3 4 5 6 7 8 9 99 1	10
13	9 97 1 2 3 4 5 6 7 8 9 98 1 2 3 4 5 6 7 8 9 99 1	11
14	9 97 1 2 4 5 6 7 8 9 98 1 2 3 4 5 6 7 8 9 99 1	12
15	9 97 1 2 3 4 5 7 8 9 98 1 2 3 4 5 6 7 8 9 99 1	13
16	9 97 1 2 4 5 6 7 8 9 98 1 2 3 4 5 6 7 8 9 99 1	14
17	9 97 2 3 4 5 6 7 8 9 98 1 2 3 4 5 6 7 8 9 99 1	15
18	9 97 1 2 4 5 6 7 8 9 98 1 2 3 4 5 6 7 8 9 99 1	16
19	9 97 2 3 4 5 6 7 8 9 98 1 2 3 4 5 6 7 8 9 99 1	17
20	9 97 1 2 3 4 5 6 7 8 9 98 1 2 3 4 5 6 7 8 9 99 1	18
21	9 97 1 2 3 4 5 6 7 8 9 98 1 2 3 4 5 6 7 8 9 99 1	19
22	9 97 1 2 3 4 5 6 7 8 9 98 1 2 3 4 5 6 7 8 9 99 1	20
23	9 97 1 2 3 4 5 6 7 8 9 98 1 2 3 4 5 6 7 8 9 99 1	21
24	9 97 1 2 3 4 5 6 7 8 9 98 1 2 3 4 5 6 7 8 9 99 1	22
25	9 97 1 2 3 4 5 6 7 8 9 98 1 2 3 4 5 6 7 8 9 99 1	23
26	9 97 1 2 3 4 5 6 7 8 9 98 1 2 3 4 5 6 7 8 9 99 1	24
27	9 97 1 2 3 4 5 6 7 8 9 98 1 2 3 4 5 6 7 8 9 99 1	25
28	9 97 1 2 3 4 5 6 7 8 9 98 1 2 3 4 5 6 7 8 9 99 1	26
29	9 97 1 2 3 4 5 6 7 8 9 98 1 2 3 4 5 6 7 8 9 99 1	27
30	9 97 1 2 3 4 5 6 7 8 9 98 1 2 3 4 5 6 7 8 9 99 1	28
31	9 97 1 2 3 4 5 6 7 8 9 98 1 2 3 4 5 6 7 8 9 99 1	29
Ap 1	9 97 1 2 3 4 5 6 7 8 9 98 1 2 3 4 5 6 7 8 9 99 1	30
2	9 97 1 2 3 4 5 6 7 8 9 98 1 2 3 4 5 6 7 8 9 99 1	31
3	9 97 1 2 3 4 5 6 7 8 9 98 1 2 3 4 5 6 7 8 9 99 1	32
4	9 97 1 2 3 4 5 6 7 8 9 98 1 2 3 4 5 6 7 8 9 99 1	33
5	9 97 1 2 3 4 5 6 7 8 9 98 1 2 3 4 5 6 7 8 9 99 1	34
6	9 97 1 2 3 4 5 6 7 8 9 98 1 2 3 4 5 6 7 8 9 99 1	

* I would like to thank Linacre Laboratories, makers of the Ovul-index (BBT) thermometer, for permission to use their charts.

across the highest of these six low temperatures.

Second. Draw another line 0.4° above the first line.

Third. Look for three *consecutive* high temperatures
(the "high set") on or above the second
line. The couple is infertile at 8:00 P.M. on
the evening this third high temperature is
recorded.

If you followed the steps properly, you will find that
the couple is infertile on Day 23. If you *didn't* calculate
accurately, follow my steps below:

1. Look for a cluster of low temperatures. (If you
turn the book sideways, it is easier to find the low
set.) There are several on Days 12 through 19. Now,
look for the six lowest *consecutive* temperatures just
before any rise begins. They occur on Days 12, 13,
14, 15, 16, and 17.

The highest of these six consecutive low temperatures is 97.7°. Draw a line along the 97.7° row of
numbers.

2. Add 0.4° to 97.7°. Answer: 98.1°. Draw a line
along the 98.1° row of numbers.

3. Now look for three consecutive temperatures
either on or above the 98.1° temperature line. They
occur on Days 21 through 23, and Day 23 is the third
in this "high set."

To see the same chart marked off as I've indicated,
look at Chart No. 1A (see page 127).

Chart No. 2. (See page 128.) There are a few small
differences in this chart. For example, the woman remembered the date of her last "menstruation." (Since the
couple wasn't previously charting temperatures, however,
they can't be sure whether the bleeding was menstrual or
intermenstrual.) The bleeding episode had begun one

Chart No. 1A

Date	Readings and Notes	
Mar 3	9 97 1 2 3 4 5 6 7 8 9 (98) 1 2 3 4 5 6 7 8 9 99 1	1
4	9 97 1 2 3 4 5 6 7 8 (9) 98 1 2 3 4 5 6 7 8 9 99 1	2
5	9 97 1 2 3 4 5 6 7 8 (9) 98 1 2 3 4 5 6 7 8 9 99 1	3
6	9 97 1 2 3 4 5 6 7 (8) 9 98 1 2 3 4 5 6 7 8 9 99 1	4
7	9 97 1 2 3 4 5 6 7 8 (9) 98 1 2 3 4 5 6 7 8 9 99 1	5
8	9 97 1 2 3 4 5 6 (7) 8 9 98 1 2 3 4 5 6 7 8 9 99 1	6
9	9 97 1 2 3 4 5 (6) 7 8 9 98 1 2 3 4 5 6 7 8 9 99 1	7
10	9 97 1 2 3 4 5 (6) 7 8 9 98 1 2 3 4 5 6 7 8 9 99 1	8
11	9 97 1 2 3 4 5 6 7 8 9 98 1 2 3 4 5 (6) 7 8 9 99 1	9
12	9 97 1 2 3 4 5 6 7 8 9 98 (2) 3 4 5 6 7 8 9 99 1	10
13	9 97 1 2 3 4 5 6 7 8 9 98 (1) 2 3 4 5 6 7 8 9 99 1	11
14	9 97 1 2 3 (4) 5 6 7 8 (9) 98 1 2 3 4 5 6 7 8 9 99 1	12
15	9 97 1 2 3 4 5 6 (7) 8 9 98 1 2 3 4 5 6 7 8 9 99 1	13
16	9 97 1 2 3 (4) 5 6 7 8 9 98 1 2 3 4 5 6 7 8 9 99 1	14
17	9 97 (3) 4 5 6 7 8 9 98 1 2 3 4 5 6 7 8 9 99 1	15
18	9 97 1 2 3 (4) 5 6 7 8 9 98 1 2 3 4 5 6 7 8 9 99 1	16
19	9 97 (2) 3 4 5 6 7 8 9/98 2 3 4 5 6 7 8 9 99 1	17
20	9 97 1 2 3 4 5 (6) 7 8 9 98 2 3 4 5 6 7 8 9 99 1	18
21	9 97 1 2 3 4 5 (6) 7 8 9 98 2 3 4 5 6 7 8 9 99 1	19
22	9 97 1 2 3 4 5 6 7 (8) 9 98 2 3 4 5 6 7 8 9 99 1	20
23	9 97 1 2 3 4 5 6 7 8 9 98 (1) 2 3 4 5 6 7 8 9 99 1	21
24	9 97 1 2 3 4 5 6 7 8 9 98 (1) 2 3 4 5 6 7 8 9 99 1	22
25	9 97 1 2 3 4 5 6 7 8 9 98 2 (3) 4 5 6 7 8 9 99 1	23
26	9 97 1 2 3 4 5 6 7 8 9 98 2 (3) 4 5 6 7 8 9 99 1	24
27	9 97 1 2 3 4 5 6 7 8 9 98 2 (3) 4 5 6 7 8 9 99 1	25
28	9 97 1 2 3 4 5 6 7 8 9 98 2 3 (4) 5 6 7 8 9 99 1	26
29	9 97 1 2 3 4 5 6 7 8 9 98 (1) 2 3 4 5 6 7 8 9 99 1	27
30	9 97 1 2 3 4 5 6 7 8 9 98 2 (4) 5 6 7 8 9 99 1	28
31	9 97 1 2 3 4 5 6 7 8 9 98 1 (2) 3 4 5 6 7 8 9 99 1	29
Apr 1	9 97 1 2 3 4 5 6 7 8 9 98 1 2 3 (4) 5 6 7 8 9 99 1	30
2	9 97 1 2 3 4 5 6 7 8 9 (98) 2 3 4 5 6 7 8 9 99 1	31
3	9 97 1 2 3 4 5 6 7 8 9 (98) 1 2 3 4 5 6 7 8 9 99 1	32
4	9 97 1 2 3 4 5 6 7 8 9 (98) 1 2 3 4 5 6 7 8 9 99 1	33
5	9 97 1 2 3 4 5 6 7 8 9 98 (1) 2 3 4 5 6 7 8 9 99 1	34
6	9 97 1 2 3 4 5 6 7 8 9 98 1 2 3 4 5 6 7 8 9 99 1	

97   98   99

Chart No. 2

*A long cycle
temperature
chart*

Date	Readings and Notes	
Aug 11	9 97 1 2 3 4 5 ⑥ 7 8 9 98 1 2 3 4 5 6 7 8 9 99 1	7
12	9 97 1 2 3 4 5 6 7 8 ⑨98 1 2 3 4 5 6 7 8 9 99 1	8
13	9 97 1 2 3 4 5 6 ⑦8 9 98 1 2 3 4 5 6 7 8 9 99 1	9
14	9 97 1 2 3 4 5 6 7 8 ⑨98 1 2 3 4 5 6 7 8 9 99 1	10
15	9 97 1 2 ③4 5 6 7 8 9 98 1 2 3 4 5 6 7 8 9 99 1	11
16	9 97 1 2 3 ④5 6 7 8 9 98 1 2 3 4 5 6 7 8 9 99 1	12
17	9 97 1 2 3 ④5 6 7 8 9 98 1 2 3 4 5 6 7 8 9 99 1	13
18	9 97 1 2 3 4 5 6 7 ⑧9 98 1 2 3 4 5 6 7 8 9 99 1	14
19	9 97 1 2 3 4 5 ⑥7 8 9 98 1 2 3 4 5 6 7 8 9 99 1	15
20	9 97 1 ②3 4 5 6 7 8 9 98 1 2 3 4 5 6 7 8 9 99 1	16
21	9 97 1 ②③4 5 6 7 8 9 98 1 2 3 4 5 6 7 8 9 99 1	17
22	9 97 1 2 3 4 ⑤6 7 8 9 98 1 2 3 4 5 6 7 8 9 99 1	18
23	9 97 1 2 ③4 5 6 7 8 9 98 1 2 3 4 5 6 7 8 9 99 1	19
24	9 97 1 2 3 4 ⑤6 7 8 9 98 1 2 3 4 5 6 7 8 9 99 1	20
25	9 97 1 2 3 4 ⑤6 7 8 9 98 1 2 3 4 5 6 7 8 9 99 1	21
26	9 97 1 2 3 ④5 6 7 8 9 98 1 2 3 4 5 6 7 8 9 99 1	22
27	9 97 1 ③4 5 6 7 8 9 98 1 2 3 4 5 6 7 8 9 99 1	23
28	9 97 1 ②4 5 6 7 8 9 98 1 2 3 4 5 6 7 8 9 99 1	24
29	9 97 1 ②4 5 6 7 8 9 98 1 2 3 4 5 6 7 8 9 99 1	25
30	9 ⑨7 1 2 3 4 5 6 7 8 9 98 1 2 3 4 5 6 7 8 9 99 1	26
31	9 97 1 ①4 5 6 7 8 9 98 1 2 3 4 5 6 7 8 9 99 1	27
Sept 1	9 97 1 ①3 4 5 6 7 8 9 98 1 2 3 4 5 6 7 8 9 99 1	28
2	9 97 1 2 ③4 5 6 7 8 9 98 1 2 3 4 5 6 7 8 9 99 1	29
3	9 97 1 2 3 4 5 6 ⑦8 9 98 1 2 3 4 5 6 7 8 9 99 1	30
4	9 97 1 2 3 4 5 6 7 8 ⑨98 1 2 3 4 5 6 7 8 9 99 1	31
5	9 97 1 2 3 4 5 6 7 8 9 98 ①2 3 4 5 6 7 8 9 99 1	32
6	9 97 1 2 3 4 5 6 7 8 9 98 ①2 3 4 5 6 7 8 9 99 1	33
7	9 97 1 2 3 4 5 6 7 8 9 98 ①2 3 4 5 6 7 8 9 99 1	34
8	9 97 1 2 3 4 5 6 7 8 9 98 ①2 3 4 5 6 7 8 9 99 1	35
9	9 97 1 2 3 4 5 6 7 8 9 98 1 ③4 5 6 7 8 9 99 1	36
10	9 97 1 2 3 4 5 6 7 8 9 98 1 2 ③4 5 6 7 8 9 99 1	37
11	9 97 1 2 3 4 5 6 7 8 9 98 1 ②3 4 5 6 7 8 9 99 1	38
12	9 97 1 2 3 4 5 6 7 8 9 98 1 2 ③4 5 6 7 8 9 99 1	39
13	9 97 1 2 3 4 5 6 7 8 9 98 1 ②3 4 5 6 7 8 9 99 1	40
14	9 97 1 2 3 4 5 6 7 8 9 ⑨98 1 2 3 4 5 6 7 8 9 99 1	41

week previously. Thus, the woman began taking her waking temperature on the morning of the seventh day of the presumed cycle.

Notice that starting on Day 23, the temperature circles are drawn in the middle, *between* two numbers—at 97.25°. This happens to be exactly where the mercury stopped, so the chart is marked to present the most accurate reading possible.

Now, follow the three steps to determine infertility:

1. Look for the six lowest consecutive temperatures.
2. Count 0.4° up from 97.25° to mark off the 0.4° separation between the low and high temperature "sets."
3. Now look for three consecutive temperatures either on the 97.65° line or above it.

The couple proves infertility by Day 32 after the third consecutive high temperature was recorded. This particular cycle lasted forty-five days, so the couple was infertile from 8:00 P.M. on Day 32 through the forty-fifth day of the cycle. Infertility lasted through at least the first six days of the succeeding cycle.

Check Chart No. 2A (see page 130) to see how the calculation was made.

Temperature disturbances: On page 121 I pointed out that you may record higher-than-normal waking temperatures if you were ill, had a few alcoholic drinks the night before and usually don't, and so on.

If you record a high temperature that is most likely caused by a disturbance, note the disturbance on your chart, *but disregard the temperature.* In other words, if you are "looking" for three high temperatures, but one of them is caused by a disturbance, ignore it. Wait until you record another high temperature without any disturbance.

Chart No. 2A

Date	Readings and Notes	
Aug 11	9 97 1 2 3 4 5 (6) 7 8 9 98 1 2 3 4 5 6 7 8 9 99 1	7
12	9 97 1 2 3 4 5 6 7 8 9 (98) 1 2 3 4 5 6 7 8 9 99 1	8
13	9 97 1 2 3 4 5 6 (7) 8 9 98 1 2 3 4 5 6 7 8 9 99 1	9
14	9 97 1 2 3 4 5 6 7 8 (9) 98 1 2 3 4 5 6 7 8 9 99 1	10
15	9 97 1 2 (5) 4 5 6 7 8 9 98 1 2 3 4 5 6 7 8 9 99 1	11
16	9 97 1 2 3 (4) 5 6 7 8 9 98 1 2 3 4 5 6 7 8 9 99 1	12
17	9 97 1 2 3 4 (5) 6 7 8 9 98 1 2 3 4 5 6 7 8 9 99 1	13
18	9 97 1 2 3 4 5 6 7 (8) 9 98 1 2 3 4 5 6 7 8 9 99 1	14
19	9 97 1 2 3 4 5 (6) 7 8 9 98 1 2 3 4 5 6 7 8 9 99 1	15
20	9 97 1 (2) 3 4 5 6 7 8 9 98 1 2 3 4 5 6 7 8 9 99 1	16
21	9 97 1 2 (3) 4 5 6 7 8 9 98 1 2 3 4 5 6 7 8 9 99 1	17
22	9 97 1 2 3 4 (5) 6 7 8 9 98 1 2 3 4 5 6 7 8 9 99 1	18
23	9 97 1 2 (3) 4 5 6 7 8 9 98 1 2 3 4 5 6 7 8 9 99 1	19
24	9 97 1 2 3 4 (5) 6 7 8 9 98 1 2 3 4 5 6 7 8 9 99 1	20
25	9 97 1 2 3 4 (3) 6 7 8 9 98 1 2 3 4 5 6 7 8 9 99 1	21
26	9 97 1 2 3 4 (3) 6 7 8 9 98 1 2 3 4 5 6 7 8 9 99 1	22
27	9 97 1 (1) 6 7 8 9 98 1 2 3 4 5 6 7 8 9 99 1	23
28	9 97 1 (1) 4 5 6 7 8 9 98 1 2 3 4 5 6 7 8 9 99 1	24
29	9 97 1 (1) 4 5 6 7 8 9 98 1 2 3 4 5 6 7 8 9 99 1	25
30	9 (97) 1 2 3 4 5 6 7 8 9 98 1 2 3 4 5 6 7 8 9 99 1	26
31	9 97 1 (1) 4 5 6 7 8 9 98 1 2 3 4 5 6 7 8 9 99 1	27
Sept 1	9 97 1 (1) 4 5 6 7 8 9 98 1 2 3 4 5 6 7 8 9 99 1	28
2	9 97 1 2 (3) 4 5 6 7 8 9 98 1 2 3 4 5 6 7 8 9 99 1	29
3	9 97 1 2 3 4 5 6 (7) 8 9 98 1 2 3 4 9 97 8 9 99 1	30
4	9 97 1 2 3 4 5 6 7 8 (9) 98 1 2 3 4 98 97 8 9 99 1	31
5	9 97 1 2 3 4 5 6 7 8 9 98 (1) 2 3 4 97 97 8 9 99 1	32
6	9 97 1 2 3 4 5 6 7 8 9 98 (1) 2 3 4 5 6 7 8 9 99 1	33
7	9 97 1 2 3 4 5 6 7 8 9 98 (1) 2 3 4 5 6 7 8 9 99 1	34
8	9 97 1 2 3 4 5 6 7 8 9 98 (1) 2 3 4 5 6 7 8 9 99 1	35
9	9 97 1 2 3 4 5 6 7 8 9 98 1 (1) 4 5 6 7 8 9 99 1	36
10	9 97 1 2 3 4 5 6 7 8 9 98 1 2 (3) 4 5 6 7 8 9 99 1	37
11	9 97 1 2 3 4 5 6 7 8 9 98 (2) 3 4 5 6 7 8 9 99 1	38
12	9 97 1 2 3 4 5 6 7 8 9 98 1 2 (3) 4 5 6 7 8 9 99 1	39
13	9 97 1 2 3 4 5 6 7 8 9 98 1 (2) 3 4 5 6 7 8 9 99 1	40
14	9 97 1 2 3 4 5 6 7 8 9 (98) 1 2 3 4 5 6 7 8 9 99 1	41

There is further information about such situations on pages 158–159. Meanwhile, the following chart will clarify most questions.

Chart No. 3. (See page 132.) This couple began charting near the end of one menstrual cycle. *They must consider the days of menstruation fertile, since the onset of the menses is not preceded by an appropriate temperature rise in this chart.* Remember: without a temperature rise, it is impossible to know for certain whether this is a true menstruation or intermenstrual bleeding. The latter may be fertile. Thus, the couple is fertile the five days of the menses (marked "M").

Try to work out the rest of this "fertility puzzle" on your own, then read below to see if you've properly proven the first day of infertility.

The couple is infertile the evening of Day 21, after 8:00 P.M.

If you didn't prove fertility on that day, follow the three steps with me:

1. Look for the six consecutive lowest temperatures before a rise begins. (Days 5, 6, 7, 8, 9, and 10.) (Note: Days 9 through 14 could also be considered.) The highest of these is 97.8°. Draw your first line along this row of temperatures.
2. Count up 0.4° from 97.8°. (97.8° plus 0.4° equals 98.2°.) Draw a line along the 98.2° row of numbers.
3. Look for three consecutive temperatures all of which are either on or above the high temperature line. (Days 18, 19, and 20.)

Ordinarily, the couple would consider themselves infertile by the evening of Day 20. However, there is a notation recorded for that day: "Drinking!" (Remember: liquor consumption can raise the waking temperature a bit, especially if you're only

Chart No. 3

Effect of liquor on temperature

Date	Readings and Notes	
Dec. 4	9 97 1 2 3 4 5 6 7 8 9 98 1 2 ③ 4 5 6 7 8 9 99 1	1
5	9 97 1 2 3 4 5 6 7 8 9 98 1 2 ⑤ 4 5 6 7 8 9 99 1	2
6	9 97 1 2 3 4 5 6 7 8 9 98 1 ② 3 4 5 6 7 8 9 99 1	3
7	9 97 1 2 3 4 5 6 7 8 9 98 1 ⓪ 4 5 6 7 8 9 99 1	4
8	9 97 1 2 3 4 5 6 7 8 9 98 1 ① 3 4 5 6 7 8 9 99 1	5
9	9 97 1 2 3 4 5 6 7 8 9 98 1 ② 3 4 5 6 7 8 9 99 1	6
10	9 97 1 2 3 4 5 6 7 8 9 98 1 ② 3 4 5 6 7 8 9 99 1	7
11	9 97 1 2 3 4 5 6 7 8 9 98 1 2 3 4 5 ⑥ 7 8 9 99 1	8
12	9 97 1 2 3 4 5 6 7 8 9 98 1 2 3 ④ 5 6 7 8 9 99 1	9
13	9 97 1 2 3 4 5 6 7 8 9 98 ① 2 3 4 5 M 8 9 99 1	1
14	9 97 1 2 3 4 5 6 7 8 9 ⑱ 1 2 3 4 5 M 8 9 99 1	2
15	9 97 1 2 3 4 5 6 7 ⑧ 9 98 1 2 3 4 5 M 8 9 99 1	3
16	9 97 1 2 3 4 5 6 7 ⑧ 9 98 1 2 3 4 5 M 8 9 99 1	4
17	9 97 1 2 3 4 ⑤ 6 7 8 9 98 1 2 3 4 5 M 8 9 99 1	5
18	9 97 1 2 3 4 5 ⑥ 7 8 9 98 1 2 3 4 5 6 7 8 9 99 1	6
19	9 97 1 2 3 4 5 6 ⑦ 8 9 98 1 2 3 4 5 6 7 8 9 99 1	7
20	9 97 1 2 3 4 5 6 ⑦ 8 9 98 1 2 3 4 5 6 7 8 9 99 1	8
21	9 97 1 2 3 4 5 6 7 ⑧ 9 98 1 2 3 4 5 6 7 8 9 99 1	9
22	9 97 1 2 3 4 5 6 ⑦ 8 9 98 1 2 3 4 5 6 7 8 9 99 1	10
23	9 97 1 2 3 4 5 6 7 ⑧ 9 98 1 2 3 4 5 6 7 8 9 99 1	11
24	9 97 1 2 3 4 5 6 7 ⑧ 9 98 1 2 3 4 5 6 7 8 9 99 1	12
25	9 97 1 2 3 4 5 6 ⑦ 8 9 98 1 2 3 4 5 6 7 8 9 99 1	13
26	9 97 1 2 3 ④ 5 6 7 8 9 98 1 2 3 4 5 6 7 8 9 99 1	14
27	9 97 1 2 3 4 5 6 7 8 ⑨ 98 1 2 3 4 5 6 7 8 9 99 1	15
28	9 97 1 2 3 4 5 6 7 ⑧ 9 98 1 2 3 4 5 6 7 8 9 99 1	16
29	9 97 1 2 3 4 5 6 7 8 9 ⑱ 1 2 3 4 5 6 7 8 9 99 1	17
30	9 97 1 2 3 4 5 6 7 8 9 98 1 ② 3 4 5 6 7 8 9 99 1	18
31	9 97 1 2 3 4 5 6 7 8 9 98 1 2 3 ④ 5 6 7 8 9 99 1	19
Jan. 1	9 97 1 *Drinking!* 98 1 2 3 4 5 6 7 8 9 ⑨⑨ 1	20
2	9 97 1 2 3 4 5 6 7 8 9 98 1 2 ③ 4 5 6 7 8 9 99 1	21
3	9 97 1 2 3 4 5 6 7 8 9 98 1 2 3 4 ⑤ 6 7 8 9 99 1	22
4	9 97 1 2 3 4 5 6 7 8 9 98 1 2 3 ④ 5 6 7 8 9 99 1	23
5	9 97 1 2 3 4 5 6 7 8 9 98 1 ② 3 4 5 6 7 8 9 99 1	24
6	9 97 1 2 3 4 5 6 7 8 9 98 1 2 ③ 4 5 6 7 8 9 99 1	25
7	9 97 1 2 3 4 5 6 7 8 9 98 1 2 3 ④ 5 6 7 8 9 99 1	26

an occasional drinker.) It happens to be January 1, the day after the New Year's Eve celebration. While recorded, *the Day 20 temperature must be ignored, since the rise may be caused by alcohol alone—not progesterone.* So in this case the couple must wait one extra day to be sure of infertility.

The couple proves that they are infertile by 8:00 P.M. on the evening of Day 21.

Additional comments. It is likely that the couple is infertile on Day 20, of course. If they were familiar with mucus and cervical changes, they could check the other signals to help determine their infertility. But since the couple is a new user of natural family planning, they must wait for the additional day of an unequivocal high temperature uninfluenced by extraneous factors. That day is Day 21.

This woman's cycle continues (though you don't see it on this chart) through Day 32. The couple is infertile through at least Day 5 of the new cycle since the menstrual/post-menstrual phase follows a sustained temperature rise. There is a greater than 99 percent likelihood that they are infertile on Day 6 of the new cycle as well.

Bleeding and the "6 and 4 and 3" guideline. If you don't notice a temperature rise and bleeding begins, *you must still consider yourselves fertile through the duration of the bleeding episode.* There is such a thing as an intermenstrual bleeding. Such a bleeding episode is *not* a true menstruation, since ovulation did not precede it. Intermenstrual bleedings may be precipitated by a drop in circulating estrogen, *not* by ovulation.

The important point is this: if you did not ovulate prior to the intermenstrual bleeding episode, it is possible to ovulate—and thus conceive—during the bleeding episode. So *unless you are checking temperatures to confirm the return of infertility, you must consider any bleeding episode to be fertile. Only* a sustained temperature rise can prove otherwise.

So for your first cycle using natural family planning, consider yourselves fertile until 8:00 P.M. on the day of the third consecutive temperature that's at least 0.4° higher than the highest temperature of the six lowest consecutive temperatures preceding the rise.

What if you don't "prove" infertility? Some couples experience shallow rises. Thus, they will not record temperatures that satisfy the requirement of the "6 and 4 and 3" guideline. In other words, they won't be able to "prove" infertility. If this happens to you, what should you do?

First, I assume, of course, that you have not been able to find NFP instruction in your area and must rely solely on the information contained in this book. Otherwise, you would, of course, consult with your teacher.

In the absence of personal counsel, fertility must be presumed *even* in the face of a shallow temperature rise if it doesn't fulfill the requirements of the "6 and 4 and 3" guideline. Fertility continues through any bleeding episode that occurs.

Obviously, you may, or may not, be in a new cycle after a bleeding episode that follows a shallow temperature rise. (Since the episode isn't defined as menstrual, the first day of bleeding can't be defined as the first day of a new cycle either.) If you feel confident that you can observe and distinguish mucus changes, you may follow the guidelines for charting the second and third cycles after a bleeding episode that follows a shallow temperature rise. If you are not confident about your ability to chart mucus, you are then "in doubt" *and fertile.* Fertility lasts until an appropriate temperature rise is recorded according to instructions that begin on page 135.

Final comment. The husband is fertile every single

day; for an indefinite time, the wife will also be "fertile" on a daily basis. It's a new situation. A great deal of couple communication, sharing, and mutual agreement is demanded. While difficult, in a very real sense, this situation is an *opportunity*.

The 21-Day Rule

Some couples rely solely on the temperature rise sign in conjunction with the so-called 21-day rule to determine the total time of infertility after ovulation. Thus, they don't chart the mucus and cervical signs.

There is a sound basis for relying on the 21-day rule. If you look at Table 3 on page 136, you will see that a couple's fertility phase begins three weeks—or 21 days—prior to the onset of menstruation. Thus, it is possible to make a highly reliable calculation of the last day of infertility beyond the sixth day. The technique? Simply subtract 21 days from the total length of the cycle.

If you look below the table, you will also see how to apply the 21-day rule in the first few cases. All you do is subtract 21 days from the last figure in the column, which is the last day of the cycle. You can also readily cross-check against the diagram to see that the calculation is accurate: the heavy black line is drawn after the last infertile day.

Test yourself by doing the calculations for the rest of the cycles. Check the results of your subtraction against the diagram: the last probable day of infertility is the figure that immediately *precedes* the black line. The results of your subtraction should yield that figure.

Applying the 21-day rule. In order to apply the rule reliably, you should have records on the lengths of *your last twelve cycles*. This improves reliability for the woman who occasionally experiences a cycle that's a day or more shorter than usual. Here's how to apply the rule:

TABLE 3: Applying the 21-Day Rule to Determine the Last Menstrual/Post-Menstrual Day of Infertility

MENSTRUAL/POST-MENSTRUAL PHASE	OVULATORY PHASE	POST-OVULATORY PHASE
Couple is infertile	Couple is fertile Conception is likely	Couple is infertile

MENSTRUAL/POST-MENSTRUAL PHASE	OVULATORY PHASE	POST-OVULATORY PHASE
1 2 3 4 5 6 7 8 9 10 11 12 13 14 15 16 17 18 19 20 21 22 23	24 25 26 27 28 29 30 31 32 33	34 35 36 37 38 39 40 41 42 43 44
1 2 3 4 5 6 7 8 9 10 11 12	13 14 15 16 17 18 19 20 21 22	23 24 25 26 27 28 29 30 31 32 33
1 2 3 4 5 6 7 8 9 10 11 12 13 14 15	16 17 18 19 20 21 22 23 24 25	26 27 28 29 30 31 32 33 34 35 36
1 2 3 4 5 6 7 8 9 10 11 12 13 14 15 16 17	18 19 20 21 22 23 24 25 26 27	28 29 30 31 32 33 34 35 36 37 38
1 2 3 4 5	6 7 8 9 10 11 12 13 14 15	16 17 18 19 20 21 22 23 24 25 26
1 2 3 4 5 6 7 8 9 10 11 12 13 14 15 16 17 18 19 20 21 22	23 24 25 26 27 28 29 30 31 32	33 34 35 36 37 38 39 40 41 42 43
1 2 3 4 5 6	7 8 9 10 11 12 13 14 15 16	17 18 19 20 21 22 23 24 25 26 27
1 2 3 4 5 6 7 8	9 10 11 12 13 14 15 16 17 18	19 20 21 22 23 24 25 26 27 28 29
1 2 3 4 5 6 7 8 9	10 11 12 13 14 15 16 17 18 19	20 21 22 23 24 25 26 27 28 29 30
1 2 3 4 5 6 7 8 9 10 11 12 13	14 15 16 17 18 19 20 21 22 23	24 25 26 27 28 29 30 31 32 33 34
1 2 3 4 5 6 7 8 9 10 11 12 13 14 15 16	17 18 19 20 21 22 23 24 25 26	27 28 29 30 31 32 33 34 35 36 37

Total length of cycle	minus (—)	21 days	equals (=)	21 Days last menstrual/post-menstrual infertile day
44	—	21	=	Day 23
33	—	21	=	Day 12
36	—	21	=	Day 15
38	—	21	=	Day 17

136

1. Look for the shortest cycle of the previous twelve.
2. Subtract 21 days from the shortest cycle you've recorded.
3. The result of your subtraction is your last probable infertile day.
4. If you ever experience a cycle shorter than any of the twelve used for applying the guideline, recalculate using the *latest* short cycle.

Effectiveness of the 21-day rule. No controlled study has been done to evaluate the reliability of the 21-day rule. But based on wide clinical experience from tens of thousands of couples in the Couple to Couple League, John and Sheila Kippley report in *The Art of Natural Family Planning* that the guideline offers about 99 percent reliability for the menstrual/post-menstrual phase. But the Kippleys emphasize that the 21-day rule *is subordinate to the appearance of mucus.*

Still, many couples rely solely on the temperature rise and the so-called 21-day rule to determine the total time of infertility after ovulation. If you have records on your previous twelve cycles, you may opt to use this simple means of determining your fertile and infertile phases. If you have complete records for only the past six to eight cycles, you can still apply the 21-day rule. Reliability, however, may be less than 99 percent.

In general, couples prefer to learn how to chart the mucus changes. So once the "6 and 4 and 3" guideline is mastered, you're ready for the next learning stage.

How to Chart the Second and Third Cycles

By charting mucus along with temperatures, you can usually extend the infertile phase *beyond* the sixth day of the new menstrual cycle. In addition, the "6 and 4 and 3" guideline can be relaxed somewhat, since you will have two fertility indicators to check against each other.

How to chart mucus changes. You are fertile all days that mucus is observed. Acts of intercourse are presumed to result in conception on these days.

If mucus develops, then disappears *without* a sustained temperature rise, *you must consider yourselves fertile for all the days that any mucus was present plus three complete dry days after its cessation.* Then if there is no mucus on the fourth day, you are infertile that evening *after* 8:00 P.M.

Here's an example: if your last day of any mucus was a Monday, you must wait for Tuesday, Wednesday, and Thursday to pass without seeing mucus. You are infertile on Friday at 8:00 P.M. (not before!) provided you saw no mucus on that day either.

Anytime you see mucus, you should mark your chart as follows:

Mark your chart with one plus sign (+) *if the mucus has one or more of the following characteristics:*

- Consistency of thick paste (yellow or white)
- Tacky
- Opaque (yellow or white)
- Thick
- If placed between thumb and forefinger, it makes tiny peaks when you separate your fingers

Mark your chart with two plus signs (++) *if the mucus has one or more of the following characteristics:*

- Consistency of creamy hand lotion
- If placed between thumb and forefinger, it remains smooth on both fingers when you separate them
- Cloudy
- Watery

- Milky
- Stretches less than one inch between two fingers
- Translucent (colorless or yellow)
- Translucent with red, brown, or pink tinge
- Sensation of wetness in the genital area ("feels wet")

Mark your chart with three plus signs (+++) *if the mucus has one or more of the following characteristics:*

- Translucent with opaque "threads" running through
- *Feels* wet
- *Feels* slippery
- *Feels* lubricative
- Looks like raw egg white
- Stretches between the fingers an inch or more

Mucus charting problems. What do you do if you've experienced "one plus sign" (+) in the morning, but by that evening you thought you felt a wet sensation (++)? Which mucus should you record?

The guideline is simple: *if you experience two types of mucus within one day, always record the more fertile of the two.*

In the above example, you would mark your chart with two plus signs (++).

Another example: if the mucus is creamy in the morning, but sticky and tacky at night, the chart should be marked with two plus signs (++) for creamy mucus.

If you're *in doubt* about two mucus types, always *assume* that you experienced the *more* fertile type. (If in doubt, you're fertile.) For example, if you weren't sure if you were wet or lubricative, *assume* that you experienced the more fertile type of mucus. Mark your chart with three plus signs (+++) for lubricative mucus.

Importance of sensation. Even without seeing mucus on your underclothes or feeling the toilet paper glide when you wipe yourself, you may feel a sensation of slipperiness and lubrication on the external genitals. In *Natural Sex,* author Mary Shivanandan reports a case of a woman who ignored sensation because she didn't *see* any mucus. The couple had relations and conceived. Thus, *it is important to be able to distinguish this slippery, lubricative sensation whether or not you can directly see the mucus.*

A slippery, lubricative *sensation* always demands a three plus (+++) indication on your chart. The quantity of mucus is not particularly important; the *quality* is. Mucus quality indicates whether or not the "channels" are open. A tiny, minuscule amount of slippery, lubricative mucus is sufficient for sperm to navigate up through the cervix. Conception could occur.

Thus, any *sensation* of slippery lubrication in the genital area is the reproductive equivalent of blazing fireworks on the Fourth of July. *This* may be the time that you are about to ovulate! *This* is the time conception is most likely to follow an act of intercourse! If you do *not* wish to conceive, do not engage in any genital-to-genital contact, including sexual intercourse.

Peak sign. The *last* day of the three-day-sign (+++) mucus is the peak. Sometimes there has been a bit of bleeding when the follicle ruptures. If so, you may detect a red, pink, or brown tinge in the mucus. This is no cause for alarm.

After the peak, when the mucus changes back to a less fertile mucus* or completely disappears, you can be-

---

* I often refer to mucus as "fertile" or "infertile." In fact, it is neither: the *woman* is fertile—not the mucus. However, I will keep to the "fertile/infertile mucus" designation because it is convenient and a widely accepted NFP colloquialism.

gin to check whether your temperatures "prove" post-ovulatory infertility.

Of course, you won't be able to tell that any particular day was the peak until after the drying-up process begins—that is, not until a whole day of drying up or dryness has been observed or felt. There may even be some mucus present, but it will revert to the cloudy, sticky, or pasty variety. At any rate, there must be *no* slippery, lubricative mucus seen or felt. If there is, you have *not* passed the mucus peak. You cannot begin to evaluate your temperatures for proof of infertility.

There is one exception: the last of any mucus observed in the menstrual/post-menstrual phase is considered "peak," and you are fertile until the evening of the fourth complete dry day after it. Incidents of mucus appearing and then disappearing can occur in long cycles where there may be intermittent patches of mucus brought on by other factors (for example, post-partum, breast-feeding). *Fertility must always be assumed during any incidence of mucus in the menstrual/post-menstrual phase because there's no sure way to know in advance whether or not ovulation will occur.*

Difficulties establishing the peak. Some women never observe any of the raw egg-white mucus or feel any slipperiness or lubricative sensation in the genital area. If this happens to you, consider the last day of *two plus* (++) mucus to be your most fertile and your peak sign.* Begin checking for a temperature rise according to the guideline given below on page 142 ("post-ovulatory infertility").

Another difficulty: almost every woman experiences situations of uncertainty. Be prepared for occasions when you think you have passed the peak (because you noticed

---

* In one study, Dr. Roetzer noted that 4.8 percent of the women were without any perceptible mucus.[2] If you discover that you belong to this small group, rely on the 21-day rule (page 135) to determine your last day of menstrual/post-menstrual infertility.

two or more "drying up" days in a row), then suddenly you feel slippery, lubricative mucus.

Your first, tentative post-peak dry days must be disregarded. You must view the last day of the *new* mucus sign as the probable peak and must begin to look for dry days again.

(Note: there may be mucus patches in the post-ovulatory phase after the temperature rises. But the sustained temperature rise indicates that there is so much progesterone in your body, that no possible ovulation can occur. That's why you don't have to worry about an unexpected return of fertility after a rise has been established. Progesterone, which causes the rise, suppresses ovulation. You can ignore any random appearances and disappearances of mucus in the post-ovulatory phase.)

Post-ovulatory infertility. This is the guideline established by Dr. Josef Roetzer to predict post-ovulatory infertility reliably:

You are infertile by 8:00 P.M. on the day that a third high waking temperature is recorded after the cessation of your most fertile mucus type. All three temperatures after mucus cessation must be higher than any six *consecutive* low temperatures recorded before a rise begins. The last of the three high readings must be at least 0.4° above *all* six of the lower temperatures.

Infertility lasts from 8:00 P.M. that evening and continues through at least Day 5 of the following cycle. According to Dr. Roetzer, the reliability of Day 6 infertility is 99.72 percent. Thus, for all practical purposes, a couple can consider themselves infertile through the sixth day of the new cycle.

Infertility continues until the first day that mucus is observed in the new cycle. After that, use the guidelines for menstrual/post-menstrual infertility, which follow below.

Menstrual/post-menstrual infertility. You are infertile on the evening of all dry days during the menstrual/post-menstrual phase. You must wait until evening because it isn't until then that the complete data about a particular day's dryness or absence of dryness are "in."

There are two exceptions to the dry-days guideline:

1. *You are fertile any day mucus is observed as well as three complete dry days after the last day that the mucus is observed. If the fourth day is also dry, you are infertile after 8:00 P.M on that day.*

For example, if you had one-plus mucus (+) on Tuesday, but are completely dry Wednesday, Thursday, and Friday, you are fertile from Tuesday straight through and including Friday. If you are dry all day on Saturday, too, you are infertile by that *evening* after 8:00 P.M.

2. *You are presumed fertile the day and night following any night or morning you had intercourse.*

For example, if you had intercourse Sunday night or Monday morning, you are fertile all day on Monday. Infertility resumes Tuesday night (when the complete data are "in") after 8:00 P.M. if that whole day (Tuesday) was dry.

(Note: *experienced* couples who can distinguish between seminal residues and developing mucus sometimes choose not to follow the alternate-day guideline during the menstrual/post-menstrual dry days. *Wait until you have relied on your fertility awareness for at least six complete cycles before you consider yourselves experienced.* Then if you are confident that you can distinguish between developing mucus and seminal fluids, you may elect to abandon this guideline.)

Special information for women with short cycles. Some women with short cycles do not experience dry days after menstruation. This is because the onset of the ovulatory phase sometimes coincides with the end of the bleeding. If you ever experience cycles shorter than twenty-six days, don't be surprised if there are no dry days when menstruation ends.

Another matter: it is possible for women with short cycles to conceive from an act of intercourse that takes place during the very last days of a prolonged menstrual bleeding, lasting longer than six days. However, the possibility of pregnancy occurring is slight. According to Dr. Roetzer's study mentioned on page 141, the possibility is less than one-half of one percent for all women.

Further charting instructions. During these next two cycles, record the mucus changes and the waking temperatures every day, beginning with the first day of your menstrual period. Later it will be possible to cut back on days of temperature taking, but don't do this until you have recorded these two complete cycles.

Other fertility observations. During these two cycles, begin checking your cervix each morning to note the changes. Do not try to record any cervical changes, just see if you can feel them. For example, do you notice the cervix feeling hard—like the tip of your nose—and then gradually developing a softer, more yielding feeling, like your lip? Do you notice that there are times when the cervix seems hard to reach, even feels *out* of reach—yet at other times is easy to touch?

Again, note these changes—don't record them—over the following two cycles. Refer to pages 177–85 for details on checking the cervix.

Some couples don't wish to learn the cervical indicators, since they are assured of effectiveness by monitoring the mucus sign and the temperature rise.

Still, some NFP instructors feel that it's a good idea to try to see if you can notice the changes over two or three cycles. This information could be helpful if you are in an atypical or unusual fertility situation, such as after childbirth or during the pre-menopause, or are highly irregular. But if you find it difficult to recognize the changes or simply don't want to learn them, rest assured that the information from the other fertility indicators will give you highly effective fertility control without any reliance on the cervix whatsoever.

Chart No. 4. (See page 146.) Look at this chart as a whole and see if you can determine the fertile and infertile phases of the cycle. I'll give you this much: the sustained temperature rise in the previous cycle proves that the first six days of this cycle are infertile.

Now try to determine:

1. The last day of menstrual/post-menstrual infertility.
2. The first day of post-ovulatory infertility.

After you've worked out both answers on your own, look below to see if you are correct. If not, read the explanation.

Last day of menstrual/post-menstrual infertility: Day 12.
First day of post-ovulatory infertility: 8:00 P.M., Day 27.

Explanation. The couple is infertile the first six days plus all the dry days from Day 7 through and including Day 12, the last day of menstrual/post-menstrual infertility.

Fertility begins with the onset of mucus on Day 13.

Chart No. 4

*A typical mucus
and tempera-
ture chart*

Date	Readings and Notes	
	9 97 1 2 3 4 5 6 7 8 9 98 1 2 3 4 5 6 M 9 99 1	1
	9 97 1 2 3 4 5 6 7 8 9 98 1 2 3 4 5 6 M 9 99 1	2
	9 97 1 2 3 4 5 6 7 8 9 98 1 2 3 4 5 6 M 9 99 1	3
	9 97 1 2 3 4 5 6 7 8 9 98 1 2 3 4 5 6 M 9 99 1	4
	9 97 1 2 3 4 5 6 7 8 9 98 1 2 3 4 5 6 M 9 99 1	5
	9 97 1 2 3 4 5 6 7 8 9 98 1 2 3 4 5 6 7 8 9 99 1	6
	9 97 1 2 3 4 5 6 7 8 9 98 1 2 3 4 5 6 7 8 9 99 1	7
	9 97 1 2 3 4 5 6 7 8 9 98 1 2 3 4 5 6 7 8 9 99 1	8
	9 97 1 2 3 4 5 6 7 8 9 98 1 2 3 4 5 6 7 8 9 99 1	9
	9 97 1 2 3 4 5 6 7 8 9 98 1 2 3 4 5 6 7 8 9 99 1	10
	9 97 1 2 3 4 5 6 7 8 9 98 1 2 3 4 5 6 7 8 9 99 1	11
	9 97 1 2 3 4 5 6 7 8 9 98 1 2 3 4 5 6 7 8 9 99 1	12
	9 97 1 2 3 4 5 6 7 8 9 98 1 2 3 4 5 6 7 8 9 99 1	13
	9 97 1 2 3 4 5 6 7 8 9 98 1 2 3 4 5 6 7 8 9 99 1	14
	9 97 1 2 3 4 5 6 7 8 9 98 1 2 3 4 5 6 7 8 9 99 1	15
	9 97 1 2 3 4 5 6 7 8 9 98 1 2 3 4 5 6 7 8 9 99 1	16
	9 97 1 2 3 4 5 6 7 8 9 98 1 2 3 4 5 6 7 8 9 99 1	17
	9 97 1 2 3 4 5 6 7 8 9 98 1 2 3 4 5 6 7 8 9 99 1	18
	9 97 1 2 3 4 5 6 7 8 9 98 1 2 3 4 5 6 7 8 9 99 1	19
	9 97 1 2 3 4 5 6 7 8 9 98 1 2 3 4 5 6 7 8 9 99 1	20
	9 97 2 3 4 5 6 7 8 9 98 1 2 3 4 5 6 7 8 9 99 1	21
	9 97 1 2 3 4 5 6 7 8 9 98 1 2 3 4 5 6 7 8 9 99 1	22
	9 97 1 2 3 4 5 7 8 9 98 1 2 3 4 5 6 7 8 9 99 1	23
	9 97 1 2 3 4 5 6 7 8 9 98 1 2 3 4 5 6 7 8 9 99 1	24
	9 97 1 2 3 4 5 6 7 8 9 98 1 2 3 4 5 6 7 8 9 99 1	25
	9 97 1 2 3 4 5 6 7 8 9 98 1 2 3 4 5 6 7 8 9 99 1	26
	9 97 1 2 3 4 5 6 7 8 9 98 1 2 3 4 5 6 7 8 9 99 1	27
	9 97 1 2 3 4 5 6 7 8 9 98 1 2 3 4 5 6 7 8 9 99 1	28
	9 97 1 2 3 4 5 6 7 8 9 98 1 2 3 4 5 6 7 8 9 99 1	29
	9 97 1 2 3 4 5 6 7 8 9 98 1 2 3 4 5 6 7 8 9 99 1	30
	9 97 1 2 3 4 5 6 7 8 9 98 1 2 3 4 5 6 7 8 9 99 1	31
	9 97 1 2 3 4 5 6 7 8 9 98 1 2 3 4 5 6 7 8 9 99 1	32
	9 97 1 2 3 4 5 6 7 8 9 98 1 2 3 4 5 6 7 8 9 99 1	33
	9 97 1 2 3 4 5 6 7 8 9 98 1 2 3 4 5 6 7 8 9 99 1	34
	9 97 1 2 3 4 5 6 7 8 9 98 1 2 3 4 5 6 7 8 9 99 1	35

Since there is no break of four complete dry days, the couple's fertility continues uninterrupted from Day 13 through the two dry days plus all the rest of the mucus days.

By Day 26, three days have passed since the cessation of the woman's most fertile mucus type, i.e., lubricative sensation noted on Days 22 and 23. If you turn the book sideways, you will see that there is a slight temperature rise after the cessation of the most fertile mucus type. Thus, it is time to evaluate the temperature to determine infertility.

1. Draw a line along the highest of the six consecutive lowest temperatures before the rise. The lowest temperatures appear on Days 13 through 22, and 97.6° is the highest of any six consecutive low temperatures just before the rise.
2. Draw a line 0.4° above 97.6°—at 98.0°.
3. Do the three temperatures after the cessation of the most fertile mucus type on Day 23 indicate a rise? They do. They are *higher* temperatures.
4. Is the last of the high temperatures at least 98.0° or higher—0.4° above the highest of the lows?

In this case the third temperature dips below the 98.0° level. The couple must wait an additional day before the last temperature recorded is 98.0° or higher. Day 27 satisfies this requirement.

The couple is infertile after 8:00 P.M. on Day 27 through Day 6 of the following cycle. Thereafter, the couple is infertile according to the guidelines for menstrual/post-menstrual infertility found on page 143.

Note: you may also mark Days 18 through 23 as the six lowest consecutive temperatures before the rise begins. If so, post-peak infertility would be proven one day later, on Day 28.

Chart No. 5. (See page 149.) This couple had a thirty-four-day cycle. They were completely infertile through Day 6 of the cycle, since menstruation followed a sustained temperature rise. Days of intercourse are circled in the menstrual/post-menstrual phase.
Determine:

1. Days of menstrual/post-menstrual infertility.
2. First day of post-ovulatory infertility.

Work out the chart on your own, then look below to see if you are correct. If not, the explanation follows.

Days of menstrual/post-menstrual infertility: Days 1 through 15, *except* Day 10 and Day 14. Those two days followed intercourse the previous evening (note the circles to indicate intercourse). The alternate days guideline applies after an act of intercourse in the menstrual/post-menstrual phase of the cycle.

First day of post-ovulatory infertility: 8:00 P.M., Day 22.

Explanation. The fertile phase begins on Day 16 when creamy mucus is observed. Day 19 is the last day of the woman's most fertile (++) mucus type. Dry days immediately follow and it is time to evaluate the waking temperatures to determine the first day of post-ovulatory infertility.

1. The highest of the six consecutive low temperatures before the rise is 97.5°. The first line is drawn along this row of temperatures.
2. The second line is drawn at 97.9°, which is 0.4° above the highest of the six lowest temperatures before the rise.
3. The three temperatures after the cessation of the most fertile mucus indicate a rise, since all three are higher temperatures.

Chart No. 5

A 34-day cycle

Date	Readings and Notes	
	9 97 1 ②3 4 5 6 7 8 9 98 1 2 3 4 5 6 7 ⁊⅄ 99 1	1
	9 97 1 2 3 4 5 6⑦8 9 98 1 2 3 4 5 6 7 ⁊⅄ 99 1	2
	9 97 1 2 3 4 5 6 7⑧9 98 1 2 3 4 5 6 7 ⁊⅄ 99 1	3
	9 97 1 2 3 4 5⑥7 8 9 98 1 2 3 4 5 6 7 ⁊⅄ 99 1	4
	9 97 1 2 3 4 5 6⑦8 9 98 1 2 3 4 5 6 7 ⁊⅄ 99 1	5
	9 97 1 2 3 4 5 6 7 8 9⑨98 1 2 3 4 5 6 7 ⁊⅄ 99 1	6
	9 97 1 2 3 4 5 6 7⑧9 98 1 2 3 4 5 6 7 8 9 99 1	7
	9 97 1 2 3 4 5 6 7 8⑨98 1 2 3 4 5 6 7 8 9 99 1	8
	9 97 1 2 3 4 5 6⑦8 9 98 1 2 3 4 5 6 7 8 9 99 1	⑨
	9 97 1 2 3④5 6 7 8 9 98 1 2 3 4 5 6 7 8 9 99 1	10
	9 97 1 2 3 4 5 6⑦8 9 98 1 2 3 4 5 6 7 8 9 99 1	11
	9 97 1 2 3 4 5⑥7 8 9 98 1 2 3 4 5 6 7 8 9 99 1	12
	9 97 1 2 3 4 5 6⑦8 9 98 1 2 3 4 5 6 7 8 9 99 1	⑬
	9 97 1 2 3④5 6 7 8 9 98 1 2 3 4 5 6 7 8 9 99 1	14
	9 97 1 2 3 4⑤6 7 8 9 98 1 2 3 4 5 6 7 8 9 99 1	15
	9 97 1 2 3 4⑤6 7 8 9 98 1 2 3 4 5 6 7 8 9 99 1	16
	9 97 1 2⑤4 5 6 7 8 9 98 1 2 3 4 5 6 7 8 9 99 1	17
	9 97 1 2 3④5 6 7 8 9 98 1 2 3 4 5 6 7 8 9 99 1	18
	9 97 1 2③4 5 6 7 8 9 98 1 2 3 4 5 6 7 8 9 99 1	19
	9 97 1 2 3 4 5 6⑦8 9 98 1 2 3 4 5 6 7 8 9 99 1	20
	9 97 1 2 3 4 5 6 7 8 9 98 ⑫3 4 5 6 7 8 9 99 1	21
	9 97 1 2 3 4 5 6 7 8 9 98 1⑫3 4 5 6 7 8 9 99 1	22
	9 97 1 2 3 4 5 6 7 8 9 98 1 2③4 5 6 7 8 9 99 1	23
	9 97 1 2 3 4 5 6 7 8 9 98 1 2 3④5 6 7 8 9 99 1	24
	9 97 1 2 3 4 5 6 7 8 9 98 1 2③4 5 6 7 8 9 99 1	25
	9 97 1 2 3 4 5 6 7 8 9 98 1 2 3 4⑤6 7 8 9 99 1	26
	9 97 1 2 3 4 5 6 7 8 9 98 1 2 3 4⑤6 7 8 9 99 1	27
	9 97 1 2 3 4 5 6 7 8 9 98 1 2③4 5 6 7 8 9 99 1	28
	9 97 1 2 3 4 5 6 7 8 9 98 1 2 3④5 6 7 8 9 99 1	29
	9 97 1 2 3 4 5 6 7 8 9 98 1 2 3 4⑤6 7 8 9 99 1	30
	9 97 1 2 3 4 5 6 7 8 9 98 1 2 3④5 6 7 8 9 99 1	31
	9 97 1 2 3 4 5 6 7 8 9 98 1 2 3④5 6 7 8 9 99 1	32
	9 97 1 2 3 4 5 6 7 8 9 98 1 2③4 5 6 7 8 9 99 1	33
	9 97 1 2 3 4 5 6 7 8 9 98 1 2③4 5 6 7 8 9 99 1	34
	9 97 1 2 3 4 5 6 7 8 9 98 1 2 3 4 5 6 7 8 9 99 1	

4. The last temperature satisfies the requirement that it be at least 0.4° above the highest of the six lowest temperatures before the rise.

The couple is infertile from 8:00 P.M. on Day 22 through Day 6 of the following cycle. Thereafter, the couple is infertile according to the guidelines for menstrual/post-menstrual infertility on page 143.

To see the same chart marked off as I have indicated, look at Chart No. 5A (see page 151).

Chart No. 6. (See page 152.) Day 1 on this chart occurs after a temperature rise in the previous cycle. Thus, the first six days are infertile. Work out the rest of the chart on your own, then check your conclusions below.

Last day of menstrual/post-menstrual infertility: Day 8.

First day of post-ovulatory infertility: 8:00 P.M., Day 21.

Explanation. Mucus begins on Day 9, and the last day of the woman's most fertile type of mucus is Day 18. By the Roetzer guideline (mucus and temperature) the couple is infertile by 8:00 P.M. on Day 21 because three high temperatures have been recorded after the cessation of the woman's most fertile mucus. Moreover, the last temperature is at least 0.4° above the highest of the six lowest temperatures before the rise.

1. Highest of six lowest temperatures just before the rise: 97.6°.
2. 0.4° above 97.6° is 98.0.
3. All three temperatures after the cessation of the woman's most fertile mucus type indicate a rise.
4. The last of the high temperatures is at least 98.0°.

Chart No. 5A

Date	Readings and Notes	
	9 97 1 ②3 4 5 6 7 8 9 98 1 2 3 4 5 6 7 ⁹⁸ 99 1	1
	9 97 1 2 3 4 5 6 ⑦8 9 98 1 2 3 4 5 6 7 ⁹⁸ 99 1	2
	9 97 1 2 3 4 5 6 7 ⑧9 98 1 2 3 4 5 6 7 ⁹⁸ 99 1	3
	9 97 1 2 3 4 5 ⑥7 8 9 98 1 2 3 4 5 6 7 ⁹⁸ 99 1	4
	9 97 1 2 3 4 5 6 ⑦8 9 98 1 2 3 4 5 6 7 ⁹⁸ 99 1	5
	9 97 1 2 3 4 5 6 7 8 9 ⑨⑧1 2 3 4 5 6 7 ⁹⁸ 99 1	6
	9 97 1 2 3 4 5 6 7 ⑧9 98 1 2 3 4 5 6 7 8 9 99 1	7
	9 97 1 2 3 4 5 6 7 8 ⑨98 1 2 3 4 5 6 7 8 9 99 1	8
	9 97 1 2 3 4 5 6 ⑦8 9 98 1 2 3 4 5 6 7 8 9 99 1	⑨
	9 97 1 2 3 ④5 6 7 8 9 98 1 2 3 4 5 6 7 8 9 99 1	10
	9 97 1 2 3 4 5 6 ⑦8 9 98 1 2 3 4 5 6 7 8 9 99 1	11
	9 97 1 2 3 4 5 ⑥7 8 9 98 1 2 3 4 5 6 7 8 9 99 1	12
	9 97 1 2 3 4 5 6 ⑦8 9 98 1 2 3 4 5 6 7 8 9 99 1	⑬
	9 97 1 2 3 ④5 6 7 8 9 98 1 2 3 4 5 6 7 8 9 99 1	14
	9 97 1 2 3 4 ⑤6 7 8 9 98 1 2 3 4 5 6 7 8 9 99 1	15
	9 97 1 2 3 4 ⑤6 7 8 9 98 1 2 3 4 5 6 7 ← ← 1	16
	9 97 1 2 ③4 5 6 7 8 9 98 1 2 3 4 5 6 7 ← ← 1	17
	9 97 1 2 3 ④5 6 7 8 9 98 1 2 3 4 5 6 7 ← ← 1	18
	9 97 1 2 ③4 5 6 7 8 98 1 2 3 4 5 6 7 ← ← 1	19
	9 97 1 2 3 4 5 6 ⑦8 98 1 2 3 4 5 6 7 8 9 99 1	20
	9 97 1 2 3 4 5 6 7 8 98 1 ②3 2 5 7 7 8 9 99 1	21
	9 97 1 2 3 4 5 6 7 8 98 1 ②3 2 5 7 7 8 9 99 1	22
	9 97 1 2 3 4 5 6 7 8 98 1 2 ③4 5 6 7 8 9 99 1	23
	9 97 1 2 3 4 5 6 7 8 98 1 2 3 ④5 6 7 8 9 99 1	24
	9 97 1 2 3 4 5 6 7 8 98 1 2 ③4 5 6 7 8 9 99 1	25
	9 97 1 2 3 4 5 6 7 8 9 98 1 2 3 4 ⑤6 7 8 9 99 1	26
	9 97 1 2 3 4 5 6 7 8 9 98 1 2 3 4 ⑤6 7 8 9 99 1	27
	9 97 1 2 3 4 5 6 7 8 9 98 1 2 ③4 5 6 7 8 9 99 1	28
	9 97 1 2 3 4 5 6 7 8 9 98 1 2 3 ④5 6 7 8 9 99 1	29
	9 97 1 2 3 4 5 6 7 8 9 98 1 2 3 4 ⑤6 7 8 9 99 1	30
	9 97 1 2 3 4 5 6 7 8 9 98 1 2 3 ④5 6 7 8 9 99 1	31
	9 97 1 2 3 4 5 6 7 8 9 98 1 2 3 ④5 6 7 8 9 99 1	32
	9 97 1 2 3 4 5 6 7 8 9 98 1 2 ③4 5 6 7 8 9 99 1	33
	9 97 1 2 3 4 5 6 7 8 9 98 1 2 ③4 5 6 7 8 9 99 1	34
	9 97 1 2 3 4 5 6 7 8 9 98 1 2 3 4 5 6 7 8 9 99 1	

Chart No. 6

A 27-day cycle

Date	Readings and Notes	
	9 97 1 2 3 4 5 6 7 8 9 98 1 2 3 4 5 6 7 99 1	1
	9 97 1 2 3 4 5 6 7 8 9 98 1 2 3 4 5 6 7 99 1	2
	9 97 1 2 3 4 5 6 7 8 9 98 1 2 3 4 5 6 7 99 1	3
	9 97 1 2 3 4 5 6 7 8 9 98 1 2 3 4 5 6 7 99 1	4
	9 97 1 2 3 4 5 6 7 8 9 98 1 2 3 4 5 6 7 99 1	5
	9 97 1 2 3 4 5 6 7 8 9 98 1 2 3 4 5 6 7 8 9 99 1	6
	9 97 1 2 3 4 5 6 7 8 9 98 1 2 3 4 5 6 7 8 9 99 1	7
	9 97 1 2 3 4 5 6 7 8 9 98 1 2 3 4 5 6 7 8 9 99 1	8
	9 97 1 2 3 4 5 6 7 8 9 98 1 2 3 4 5 6 7 99 1	9
	9 97 1 2 3 4 5 6 7 8 9 98 1 2 3 4 5 6 7 8 9 99 1	10
	9 97 1 2 3 4 5 6 7 8 9 98 1 2 3 4 5 6 7 8 9 99 1	11
	9 97 1 2 3 4 5 6 7 8 9 98 1 2 3 4 5 6 7 8 9 99 1	12
	9 97 1 2 3 4 5 6 7 8 9 98 1 2 3 4 5 99 1	13
	9 97 1 2 3 4 5 6 7 8 9 98 1 2 3 4 5 99 1	14
	9 97 1 2 3 4 5 6 7 8 9 98 1 2 3 4 5 99 1	15
	9 97 1 2 3 4 5 6 7 8 9 98 1 2 3 4 5 6 99 1	16
	9 97 1 2 3 4 5 6 7 8 9 98 1 2 3 4 5 6 99 1	17
	9 97 1 2 3 4 5 6 7 8 9 98 1 2 3 4 5 6 99 1	18
	9 97 1 2 3 4 5 6 7 8 9 98 1 2 3 4 5 6 7 8 9 99 1	19
	9 97 1 2 3 4 5 6 7 8 9 98 1 2 3 4 5 6 7 99 1	20
	9 97 1 2 3 4 5 6 7 8 9 98 1 2 3 4 5 6 7 8 9 99 1	21
	9 97 1 2 3 4 5 6 7 8 9 98 1 2 3 4 5 6 7 8 9 99 1	22
	9 97 1 2 3 4 5 6 7 8 9 98 1 2 3 4 5 6 7 8 9 99 1	23
	9 97 1 2 3 4 5 6 7 8 9 98 1 2 3 4 5 6 7 8 9 99 1	24
	9 97 1 2 3 4 5 6 7 8 9 98 1 2 3 4 5 6 7 8 9 99 1	25
	9 97 1 2 3 4 5 6 7 8 9 98 1 2 3 4 5 6 7 8 9 1	26
	9 97 1 2 3 4 5 6 7 8 9 98 1 2 3 4 5 6 7 8 9 99 1	27
	9 97 1 2 3 4 5 6 7 8 9 98 1 2 3 4 5 6 7 8 9 99 1	
	9 97 1 2 3 4 5 6 7 8 9 98 1 2 3 4 5 6 7 8 9 99 1	
	9 97 1 2 3 4 5 6 7 8 9 98 1 2 3 4 5 6 7 8 9 99 1	
	9 97 1 2 3 4 5 6 7 8 9 98 1 2 3 4 5 6 7 8 9 99 1	
	9 97 1 2 3 4 5 6 7 8 9 98 1 2 3 4 5 6 7 8 9 99 1	
	9 97 1 2 3 4 5 6 7 8 9 98 1 2 3 4 5 6 7 8 9 99 1	
	9 97 1 2 3 4 5 6 7 8 9 98 1 2 3 4 5 6 7 8 9 99 1	
	9 97 1 2 3 4 5 6 7 8 9 98 1 2 3 4 5 6 7 8 9 99 1	

Infertility lasts from 8:00 P.M. on Day 21 through the first six days of the succeeding cycle.

Thereafter, the guidelines for menstrual/post-menstrual infertility apply.

Chart No. 7. (See page 154.) This couple is infertile for the first six days in this cycle since it follows a temperature rise in the previous cycle. Again, work out on a day-by-day basis when infertility ends and when it resumes again. After you've worked out the chart on your own, check the answers below.

Last day of menstrual/post-menstrual infertility: Day 12.

First day of post-ovulatory infertility: After 8:00 P.M., Day 21.

Explanation. Infertility lasts through Day 12 because all days are dry.

Post-ovulatory infertility is determined according to the Roetzer mucus and temperature guideline. The most fertile mucus ceases on Day 18 and a temperature rise is observed thereafter. To apply the guideline, check the following:

1. Highest of six lowest temperatures before the rise: 97.6°.
2. 0.4° above 97.6° is 98.0.
3. All three temperatures after the cessation of the most fertile mucus type are high.
4. The third high temperature after the cessation of the mucus is 98.0°.

Infertility lasts from 8:00 P.M. on Day 21 through Day 6 of the following cycle. Thereafter, infertility continues according to the guidelines for menstrual/post-menstrual infertility.

Chart No. 7

A 31-day cycle

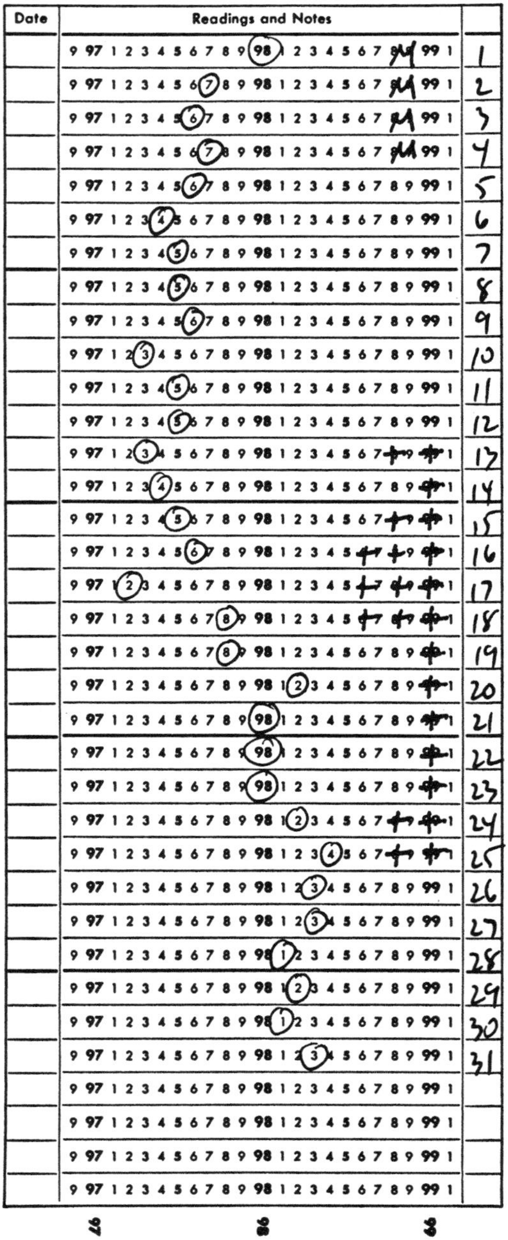

When Your Chart Doesn't Fit the Guidelines

Speaking at the International Symposium on Natural Family Planning conducted at the Human Life Center at St. John's University in Collegeville, Minnesota, in June of 1977, Dr. Roetzer made a cautionary comment about his guideline: "[The guideline] is sufficient for almost all cases; there are only a few cases where you cannot apply this rule; and there is NO rule which is appropriate for ALL cases."

Dr. Roetzer's cautionary comment is important to remember, since every couple occasionally experiences cycles that either don't meet the guidelines or are hard to interpret.* In such situations, of course, the "if in doubt, you're fertile" rule is applicable. If it is important to avoid pregnancy, defer intercourse until infertility can definitely be proven.

Of course, this is where experience will stand you in good stead. There may be times when you will have to discuss the guidelines, try to understand what has gone on, and then make a determination as to whether or not you are fertile or infertile at a particular time. Chart No. 8 demonstrates this difficulty, and shows how the couple coped with it.

Chart No. 8. (See page 156.) This couple is infertile through Day 6, since this cycle follows one in which there was a sustained temperature rise. Infertility continues through Day 9.

Mucus begins on Day 10; the couple is fertile from Day 10 through Day 16, when the woman's most fertile mucus type ceases. This couple is still fertile on Day 17 and Day 18 when there is only a yellow, tacky mucus; on

---

* The Huneger translation of Dr. Roetzer's own book on NFP is very useful. For information on obtaining the book, see Appendix C.

Chart No. 8

A shallow temperature rise

Date	Readings and Notes	
	9 97 1 2 3 4 5 6 7 ⑧ 9 98 1 2 3 4 5 6 7 8 9 99 1	1
	9 97 1 2 3 4 5 ⑥ 8 9 98 1 2 3 4 5 6 7 8 9 99 1	2
	9 97 1 2 3 4 5 6 ⑦ 8 9 98 1 2 3 4 5 6 7 8 9 99 1	3
	9 97 1 2 3 4 5 6 7 ⑧ 9 98 1 2 3 4 5 6 7 8 9 99 1	4
	9 97 1 2 3 4 5 6 ⑦ 8 9 98 1 2 3 4 5 6 7 8 9 99 1	5
	9 97 1 2 3 4 5 6 ⑦ 8 9 98 1 2 3 4 5 6 7 8 9 99 1	6
	9 97 1 2 3 4 5 6 7 ⑧ 9 98 1 2 3 4 5 6 7 8 9 99 1	7
	9 97 1 2 3 4 ⑤ 6 7 8 9 98 1 2 3 4 5 6 7 8 9 99 1	8
	9 97 1 2 3 4 5 6 ⑦ 8 9 98 1 2 3 4 5 6 7 8 9 99 1	9
	9 97 1 2 3 ④ 5 6 7 8 9 98 1 2 3 4 5 6 7 8 9 99 1	10
	9 97 1 2 3 4 ⑤ 6 7 8 9 98 1 2 3 4 5 6 7 8 9 99 1	11
	9 97 1 2 3 ④ 5 6 7 8 9 98 1 2 3 4 5 6 7 8 9 99 1	12
	9 97 1 2 3 ⑤ 6 7 8 9 98 1 2 3 4 5 6 7 8 9 99 1	13
	9 97 1 2 3 4 ⑤ 6 7 8 9 98 1 2 3 4 5 6 7 8 9 99 1	14
	9 97 1 2 3 4 5 ⑥ 7 8 9 98 1 2 3 4 5 6 7 8 9 99 1	15
	9 97 1 2 3 4 5 ⑥ 7 8 9 98 1 2 3 4 5 6 7 8 9 99 1	16
	9 97 1 2 3 4 ⑤ 6 7 8 9 98 1 2 3 4 5 6 7 8 9 99 1	17
	9 97 1 2 3 4 5 ⑥ 7 8 9 98 1 2 3 4 5 6 7 8 9 99 1	18
	9 97 1 2 3 4 5 6 ⑦ 8 9 98 1 2 3 4 5 6 7 8 9 99 1	19
	9 97 1 2 3 4 5 6 7 ⑧ 9 98 1 2 3 4 5 6 7 8 9 99 1	20
	9 97 1 2 3 4 5 6 7 ⑧ 9 98 1 2 3 4 5 6 7 8 9 99 1	21
	9 97 1 2 3 4 5 6 7 8 ⑨ 98 1 2 3 4 5 6 7 8 9 99 1	22
	9 97 1 2 3 4 5 6 7 8 ⑨ 98 1 2 3 4 5 6 7 8 9 99 1	23
	9 97 1 2 3 4 5 6 7 8 ⑨ 98 1 2 3 4 5 6 7 8 9 99 1	24
	9 97 1 2 3 4 5 6 7 8 ⑨ 98 1 2 3 4 5 6 7 8 9 99 1	25
	9 97 1 2 3 4 5 6 7 ⑧ 9 98 1 2 3 4 5 6 7 8 9 99 1	26
	9 97 1 2 3 4 5 6 7 8 ⑨ 98 1 2 3 4 5 6 7 8 9 99 1	27
	9 97 1 2 3 4 5 6 7 8 9 ⑨⑧ 1 2 3 4 5 6 7 8 9 99 1	28
	9 97 1 2 3 4 5 6 7 8 ⑨ 98 1 2 3 4 5 6 7 8 9 99 1	29
	9 97 1 2 3 4 5 6 7 8 9 98 1 2 3 4 5 6 7 8 9 99 1	
	9 97 1 2 3 4 5 6 7 8 9 98 1 2 3 4 5 6 7 8 9 99 1	
	9 97 1 2 3 4 5 6 7 8 9 98 1 2 3 4 5 6 7 8 9 99 1	
	9 97 1 2 3 4 5 6 7 8 9 98 1 2 3 4 5 6 7 8 9 99 1	
	9 97 1 2 3 4 5 6 7 8 9 98 1 2 3 4 5 6 7 8 9 99 1	
	9 97 1 2 3 4 5 6 7 8 9 98 1 2 3 4 5 6 7 8 9 99 1	

Day 19 the woman is dry. When is the couple definitely infertile again?

The answer isn't clear.

Look at the temperatures. The six lowest occur on Days 10 through 15; the highest of the lows is 97.6°. Adding 0.4° to that, the third temperature after the cessation of the woman's most fertile mucus type must reach 98.0° or higher. But no temperature achieves this level until Day 28, the second to last day of the cycle. Does this mean that the couple must wait until that day before they are infertile again?

No, it doesn't, but it does require that the couple consider their chart together very carefully.

In this case, there is a very slight temperature rise, but no dramatic rise. However, two temperatures are just .05° below the required high level—temperature 97.95° on Days 22 and 23.

The couple decided to consider themselves infertile by Day 22. Here are their reasons:

1. The couple is experienced. This is their ninth charted cycle.

2. Past charts have shown a shallow temperature rise. The couple concluded that shallow rises are typical for the wife. She has always had one temperature 0.4° above the highest of the six lowest temperatures by at least the fourth day after the cessation of the most fertile mucus. Moreover, sometimes there were only two or three temperatures that were this high in the postovulatory phase.

3. Apart from the temperature indicator, Day 22 marks the *fourth* completely dry day after the cessation of all mucus, including the one-plus (+) tacky mucus.

In the light of their past experience, this couple considers these factors—a shallow temperature rise and four completely dry days—sufficient indication that they are certainly infertile after 8:00 P.M. on Day 22. The onset of menstruation nine days later confirms the fact that ovulation probably occurred around Day 14, 15, or 16. Thus, their calculation of infertility was well within the proper range.

What to do about fevers. Disregard any temperature caused by fever. *Be especially alert to very mild fevers. Flu or a cold may cause only a slight rise of two- or three-tenths of a degree.* You could mistake these temperatures for the beginning of a rise, but such temperatures would be a *false rise.*

Do *not* use your BBT thermometer if you know you have a high temperature. The temperature will not accurately reflect your fertility or infertility anyway. Instead, use a regular fever thermometer and note the fact that you are sick on your chart.

If you have a shallow rise accompanied by flu or cold symptoms, record the rise but note that you are sick. *Do not rely on higher temperatures that are recorded when you are sick.*

Consider yourselves fertile until any possible cold, flu, or fever temperature has been gone for three full days. After the three days have passed, evaluate your chart very carefully to check that all the other infertility signs are present.

Unusually high temperatures. Very high temperatures in the menstrual/post-menstrual phase can present a different problem. Determining the highest of your lowest six consecutive temperatures would be difficult if one temperature towers way above the rest in the set. Should that happen, you would be forced to draw a line that's so high none of the later post-ovulatory high temperatures could satisfy the requirements to prove infertility.

What do you do?

First, you can always completely discount one unexpected high temperature in the menstrual/post-menstrual phase. Such unexpected highs occur from time to time and can be safely ignored if they appear among a cluster of five other low temperatures. Thus, cancel the unexpected high temperature in your calculations.

Still, any sudden temperature rise of 0.5° or more in one day is suspect. It can be ignored, of course, if it appears among the six lowest menstrual/post-menstrual temperatures. *But a sudden high temperature can never be ignored if it is one of the three high post-ovulatory temperatures. You must wait for one more (i.e., a fourth) confirmatory high temperature.*

Chart No. 9. (See page 160.) This chart begins after a temperature rise is recorded for the previous cycle. Thus, the couple is infertile for the first six days of the new cycle. Now determine:

1. The last day of menstrual/post-menstrual infertility.
2. The first day of post-ovulatory infertility.

After you've worked out both answers on your own, look below to see if you are correct. The explanation follows.

Last day of menstrual/post-menstrual infertility: Day 8.

First day of post-ovulatory infertility: Day 22.

Explanation. The chart shows an unusually high temperature of 98.0° on Day 15. The six temperatures before Day 15 are 97.6° or less; the two temperatures after Day 15 are also 97.6° or less. The temperature on Day 15 can be canceled, ignored. After the cancellation is made, the Roetzer guideline can be applied. The most fertile mucus ceases on Day 19 and a temperature rise is observed.

1. Highest of the six lowest temperatures (excluding the canceled temperature on Day 15) is 97.6°.

Chart No. 9

*An unusually
high tempera-
ture*

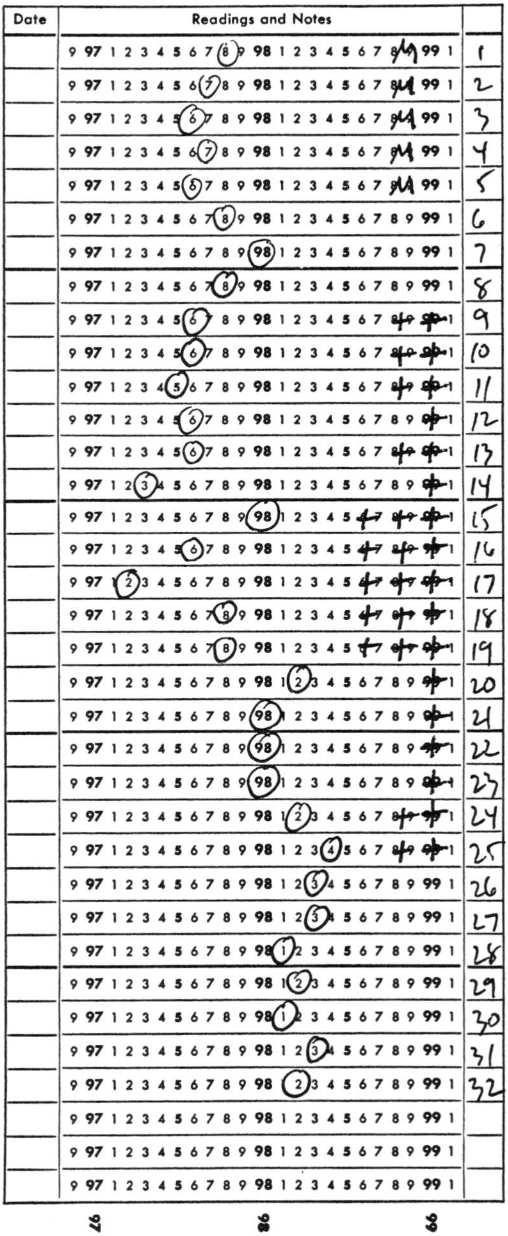

2. 0.4° above 97.6° is 98.0.

3. All three temperatures after the cessation of the most fertile type of mucus are high.

4. The last high temperature (98.0°) is 0.4° above the highest of the six consecutive low temperatures (97.6°).

Infertility lasts from 8:00 P.M. on Day 22 through Day 6 of the succeeding cycle. Thereafter, infertility will continue according to the menstrual/post-menstrual infertility guidelines.

Double jeopardy. What if you have *two* unexpected high temperatures in what you were hoping could be your set of six consecutive low temperatures?

This is where a trained instructor can offer guidance. In general, you can disregard two unusually high temperatures if there are extraneous factors that explain the unexpected highs *and* if there is an appropriate sustained temperature rise after the cessation of the woman's fertile mucus.

What "extraneous factors" are sufficient to discount the unexpected highs? These are most common:

• Cold or flu symptoms.
• Consuming alcohol the night before when you usually don't.
• Sleeping unusually late.
• Experiencing an unaccustomed chill or heat. (One couple began using an electric blanket and the wife's waking temperature rose for several consecutive days. The couple finally realized that the extra warmth from the blanket was affecting her waking temperature. From then on, all temperature taking took into account whether or not the couple used the blanket.)

If you discount two temperatures in the menstrual/ post-menstrual phase for extraneous reasons, consider yourselves fertile for one extra day of high temperatures in the post-ovulatory phase. The temperature on this extra day must be 0.4° above the highest of the menstrual/post-menstrual lows that you are considering.

Chart No. 10. (See page 163.) This chart reflects two interpretive difficulties:

> 1. The woman has short cycles and thus has difficulty establishing six consecutive low temperatures in the menstrual/post-menstrual phase. As a result, the highest of any six temperatures may be so high that it may be impossible to determine the post-ovulatory higher temperature phase according to the guidelines.
> 2. A shallow temperature rise.

With these two interpretive difficulties, the couple determines that Day 17 at 8:00 P.M. is their first post-ovulatory infertile day. Here's their reasoning:

> 1. The couple determined that Days 3 through 8 were their six low-temperature days. They canceled the temperature on Day 3 to establish 97.9° as the high for those six days.
> 2. While shallow, there *is* a temperature rise that begins with the onset of fertile-time mucus. The most fertile mucus secretion ends on Day 13. The temperatures are 98.1° or 98.2° on Days 14, 15, and 16. The last temperature, however, doesn't satisfy the requirement that it be 0.4° above the highest of the six low temperatures before the rise. In this case, the couple would be looking for a temperature of at least 98.3°.
> 3. The couple decides that their rise is shallow—a maximum of 0.3° rather than 0.4°—but that it definitely *is* a rise. Moreover, this is their third charted

Chart No. 10

*A short cycle
with shallow
rise*

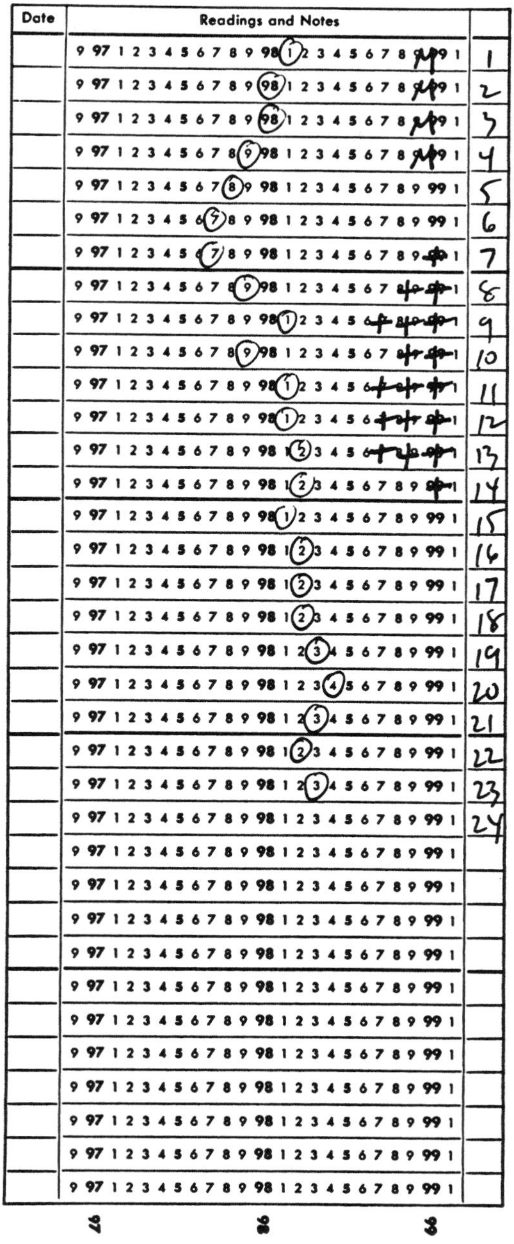

cycle and in each of the first two cycles a shallow rise was also recorded. The couple waits *four* days after the cessation of the most fertile type of mucus—rather than three days—to insure that the shallow rise is sustained. It is. Thus, they consider themselves fertile on Day 17.

The onset of menstruation nine days later proves that the couple was within the proper range.

Check Chart No. 10A (see page 165) to see how the couple marked it.

Chart No. 11. (See page 166.) Here there is a rising trend recorded after the cessation of the fertile mucus. However, the third temperature after the cessation of the most fertile mucus drops *below* the highest of the six previous temperatures just before the rise begins.*

This kind of pattern shows up cycle after cycle in a few individual women. In such cases, one low temperature among the three post-mucus peak temperatures can be ignored, but the last temperature—the fourth—must be 0.4° above the highest of those six lowest temperatures just before the rise begins.

In this case, the low temperature on Day 18 is ignored. The couple is fertile from Day 10 (first day of mucus) until 8:00 P.M. on Day 19.

Free Pregnancy Evaluation

Only complete abstinence offers 100 percent assurance that pregnancy won't occur. Selective abstinence based on the couple's correct identification of the fertile and infertile phases offers 99.2 percent reliability. The combination Pill and surgical sterilization can also offer this reliability, but with health risks.

---

* See the Huneger translation of Roetzer's guidelines for more information about "temperature drop" charts. See Appendix C for information on obtaining the book.

Chart No. 10A

A short cycle with shallow rise

Date	Readings and Notes	
	9 97 1 2 3 4 5 6 7 8 9 98 ①2 3 4 5 6 7 8 9 99 1	1
	9 97 1 2 3 4 5 6 7 8 9 ㉚1 2 3 4 5 6 7 8 99 1	2
	9 97 1 2 3 4 5 6 7 8 ㉚1 2 ⑥5 6 7 8 99 1	3
	9 97 1 2 3 4 5 6 7 ⑧98 1 2 ⑤5 6 7 8 99 1	4
	9 97 1 2 3 4 5 6 7 ⑧ 98 1 2 ④5 6 7 8 9 99 1	5
	9 97 1 2 3 4 5 ⑦8 9 98 1 2 ③5 6 7 8 9 99 1	6
	9 97 1 2 3 4 5 6 ⑦8 9 98 1 2 3②5 6 7 8 9 99 1	7
	9 97 1 2 3 4 5 6 7 ①98 1 2 3 4 5 6 7 99 99 1	8
	9 97 1 2 3 4 5 6 7 8 9 98①2 3 4 5 6 7 99 99 1	9
	9 97 1 2 3 4 5 6 7 8 ⑨98 1 2 3 4 5 6 7 99 99 1	10
	9 97 1 2 3 4 5 6 7 8 9 98①2 3 4 5 6 7 99 99 1	11
	9 97 1 2 3 4 5 6 7 8 9 98①2 3 4 5 6 7 99 99 1	12
	9 97 1 2 3 4 5 6 7 8 9 98 1②3 4 5 6 7 99 99 1	13
	9 97 1 2 3 4 5 6 7 8 9 98 1②3 4 5 ⑥7 8 9 99 1	14
	9 97 1 2 3 4 5 6 7 8 9 98①2 3 4 5②6 7 8 9 99 1	15
	9 97 1 2 3 4 5 6 7 8 9 98 1②3 4 ②7 8 9 99 1	16
	9 97 1 2 3 4 5 6 7 8 9 98 1②3 4 ④7 8 9 99 1	17
	9 97 1 2 3 4 5 6 7 8 9 98 1②3 4 5 6 7 8 9 99 1	18
	9 97 1 2 3 4 5 6 7 8 9 98 1 2③4 5 6 7 8 9 99 1	19
	9 97 1 2 3 4 5 6 7 8 9 98 1 2 3④5 6 7 8 9 99 1	20
	9 97 1 2 3 4 5 6 7 8 9 98 1 2③4 5 6 7 8 9 99 1	21
	9 97 1 2 3 4 5 6 7 8 9 98 1②3 4 5 6 7 8 9 99 1	22
	9 97 1 2 3 4 5 6 7 8 9 98 1 2③4 5 6 7 8 9 99 1	23
	9 97 1 2 3 4 5 6 7 8 9 98 1 2 3 4 5 6 7 8 9 99 1	24
	9 97 1 2 3 4 5 6 7 8 9 98 1 2 3 4 5 6 7 8 9 99 1	
	9 97 1 2 3 4 5 6 7 8 9 98 1 2 3 4 5 6 7 8 9 99 1	
	9 97 1 2 3 4 5 6 7 8 9 98 1 2 3 4 5 6 7 8 9 99 1	
	9 97 1 2 3 4 5 6 7 8 9 98 1 2 3 4 5 6 7 8 9 99 1	
	9 97 1 2 3 4 5 6 7 8 9 98 1 2 3 4 5 6 7 8 9 99 1	
	9 97 1 2 3 4 5 6 7 8 9 98 1 2 3 4 5 6 7 8 9 99 1	
	9 97 1 2 3 4 5 6 7 8 9 98 1 2 3 4 5 6 7 8 9 99 1	
	9 97 1 2 3 4 5 6 7 8 9 98 1 2 3 4 5 6 7 8 9 99 1	
	9 97 1 2 3 4 5 6 7 8 9 98 1 2 3 4 5 6 7 8 9 99 1	
	9 97 1 2 3 4 5 6 7 8 9 98 1 2 3 4 5 6 7 8 9 99 1	
	9 97 1 2 3 4 5 6 7 8 9 98 1 2 3 4 5 6 7 8 9 99 1	

97   98   99

Chart No. 11

A temperature drop

Date	Readings and Notes	
	9 97 1 2 3 4 5 6 7⑧9 98 1 2 3 4 5 6 7 8 99 1	1
	9 97 1 2 3 4 5 6⑦8 9 98 1 2 3 4 5 6 7 8 99 1	2
	9 97 1 2 3 4 5 6 7⑧9 98 1 2 3 4 5 6 7 8 99 1	3
	9 97 1 2 3 4 5 6⑦8 9 98 1 2 3 4 5 6 7 8 99 1	4
	9 97 1 2 3 4 5 6⑦8 9 98 1 2 3 4 5 6 7 8 9 99 1	5
	9 97 1 2 3 4 5⑥7 8 9 98 1 2 3 4 5 6 7 8 9 99 1	6
	9 97 1 2 3 4 5 6⑦8 9 98 1 2 3 4 5 6 7 8 9 99 1	7
	9 97 1 2 3 4 5⑥7 8 9 98 1 2 3 4 5 6 7 8 9 99 1	8
	9 97 1 2 3④5 6 7 8 9 98 1 2 3 4 5 6 7 8 9 99 1	9
	9 97 1 2 3 4 5⑥7 8 9 98 1 2 3 4 5 6 7 99 1	10
	9 97 1 2 3 4 5⑥7 8 9 98 1 2 3 4 5 6 7 99 1	11
	9 97 1 2 3 4 5 6⑦8 9 98 1 2 3 4 5 6 7 99 1	12
	9 97 1 2 3 4 5 6⑦8 9 98 1 2 3 4 5 6 99 1	13
	9 97 1 2 3 4 5⑥7 8 9 98 1 2 3 4 5 6 99 1	14
	9 97 1 2 3 4 5 6 7⑧9 98 1 2 3 4 5 6 99 1	15
	9 97 1 2 3 4 5 6 7 8⑨98 1 2 3 4 5 6 7 99 1	16
	9 97 1 2 3 4 5 6 7 8 9⑨98 1 2 3 4 5 6 7 8 9 99 1	17
	9 97 1 2 3 4 5⑥7 8 9 98 1 2 3 4 5 6 7 8 9 99 1	18
	9 97 1 2 3 4 5 6 7 8 9 98⑫3 4 5 6 7 8 9 99 1	19
	9 97 1 2 3 4 5 6 7 8 9 98⑪2 3 4 5 6 7 8 9 99 1	20
	9 97 1 2 3 4 5 6 7 8 9 98 1⑫3 4 5 6 7 8 9 99 1	21
	9 97 1 2 3 4 5 6 7 8 9 98⑪2 3 4 5 6 7 8 9 99 1	22
	9 97 1 2 3 4 5 6 7 8 9 98⑪2 3 4 5 6 7 8 9 99 1	23
	9 97 1 2 3 4 5 6 7 8 9 98 1⑫3 4 5 6 7 8 9 99 1	24
	9 97 1 2 3 4 5 6 7 8 9⑨8 1 2 3 4 5 6 7 8 9 99 1	25
	9 97 1 2 3 4 5 6 7 8 9⑨8 1 2 3 4 5 6 7 8 9 99 1	26
	9 97 1 2 3 4 5 6 7 8 9 98⑪2 3 4 5 6 7 8 9 99 1	27
	9 97 1 2 3 4 5 6 7 8 9 98 1⑫3 4 5 6 7 8 9 99 1	28
	9 97 1 2 3 4 5 6 7 8 9 98⑪2 3 4 5 6 7 8 9 99 1	29
	9 97 1 2 3 4 5 6 7 8 9⑨8 2 3 4 5 6 7 8 9 99 1	30
	9 97 1 2 3 4 5 6 7 8 9 98 1 2 3 4 5 6 7 8 9 99 1	
	9 97 1 2 3 4 5 6 7 8 9 98 1 2 3 4 5 6 7 8 9 99 1	
	9 97 1 2 3 4 5 6 7 8 9 98 1 2 3 4 5 6 7 8 9 99 1	
	9 97 1 2 3 4 5 6 7 8 9 98 1 2 3 4 5 6 7 8 9 99 1	
	9 97 1 2 3 4 5 6 7 8 9 98 1 2 3 4 5 6 7 8 9 99 1	

Should you become pregnant following Dr. Roetzer's guidelines, Dr. Roetzer would like the opportunity to study your charts. He asks, however, that such a pregnancy be *truly unexplained.* That is, that the couple have kept to the guidelines, refraining from all fertile-time sexual contact, including genital-to-genital contact without penetration. Please send *all* your original charts beginning with your *first* day of charting. (All charts will be returned, so do not send photocopies.) Be sure that your name is on *each* chart and your name and address are clearly written on a covering letter. Send the material to:

Dr. Josef Roetzer
c/o The Human Life Center
St. John's University
Collegeville, Minn. 56321

Please allow eight to twelve weeks for reply.

Do-it-yourselves Charts

The next three charts are blank. Use them to chart three practice cycles. Use the information listing the temperature and mucus signs for each cycle day. Fill in the chart appropriately. As you do so, determine fertility and infertility *for each day* and note the following:

1. The menstrual/post-menstrual infertile days,
2. The fertile days,
3. The first post-ovulatory infertile day.

At the bottom of each page you will find the three answers plus any extra commentary necessary to explain the answer. Don't peek until you've figured out the chart on your own!

Chart No. 12. (See page 169.)

Day 1:	Menstruation (M) following a sustained temperature rise in previous cycle. 98.1°	Day 12: Raw-egg-white mucus. 98.0°
Day 2:	Menstruation. 98.0°	Day 13: Tacky mucus. 97.8°
Day 3:	Menstruation. 97.8°	Day 14: Tacky mucus. 98.0°

Day 1: Menstruation
(M) following a
sustained tempera-
ture rise in pre-
vious cycle. 98.1°

Day 2: Menstruation.
98.0°

Day 3: Menstruation.
97.8°

Day 4: Menstruation.
97.8°

Day 5: Menstruation.
97.7°

Day 6: Dry. 97.6°

Day 7: Wet sensation.
97.4°

Day 8: Tacky mucus.
97.5°

Day 9: Tacky mucus.
97.5°

Day 10: Wet sensation.
97.4°

Day 11: Lubricative sensation. 97.6°

Day 12: Raw-egg-white
mucus. 98.0°

Day 13: Tacky mucus.
97.8°

Day 14: Tacky mucus.
98.0°

Day 15: Tacky, yellow
mucus. 98.6°

Day 16: Tacky, yellow
mucus. 98.3°

Day 17: Wet sensation.
98.4°

Day 18: Dry. 98.2°

Day 19: Dry. 98.4°

Day 20: Dry. 98.4°

Day 21: Dry. 98.5°

Day 22: Dry. 98.3°

Day 23: Dry. 98.5°

Day 24: Dry. 98.4°

Day 25: Dry. 98.4°

Day 26: Dry. 98.3°

Day 27: Dry. 98.3

Infertile: Through Day 6
Fertile: Day 7 through Day 14
Infertile: 8:00 P.M., Day 15

Chart No. 12

Date	Readings and Notes	
	9 97 1 2 3 4 5 6 7 8 9 98 1 2 3 4 5 6 7 8 9 99 1	
	9 97 1 2 3 4 5 6 7 8 9 98 1 2 3 4 5 6 7 8 9 99 1	
	9 97 1 2 3 4 5 6 7 8 9 98 1 2 3 4 5 6 7 8 9 99 1	
	9 97 1 2 3 4 5 6 7 8 9 98 1 2 3 4 5 6 7 8 9 99 1	
	9 97 1 2 3 4 5 6 7 8 9 98 1 2 3 4 5 6 7 8 9 99 1	
	9 97 1 2 3 4 5 6 7 8 9 98 1 2 3 4 5 6 7 8 9 99 1	
	9 97 1 2 3 4 5 6 7 8 9 98 1 2 3 4 5 6 7 8 9 99 1	
	9 97 1 2 3 4 5 6 7 8 9 98 1 2 3 4 5 6 7 8 9 99 1	
	9 97 1 2 3 4 5 6 7 8 9 98 1 2 3 4 5 6 7 8 9 99 1	
	9 97 1 2 3 4 5 6 7 8 9 98 1 2 3 4 5 6 7 8 9 99 1	
	9 97 1 2 3 4 5 6 7 8 9 98 1 2 3 4 5 6 7 8 9 99 1	
	9 97 1 2 3 4 5 6 7 8 9 98 1 2 3 4 5 6 7 8 9 99 1	
	9 97 1 2 3 4 5 6 7 8 9 98 1 2 3 4 5 6 7 8 9 99 1	
	9 97 1 2 3 4 5 6 7 8 9 98 1 2 3 4 5 6 7 8 9 99 1	
	9 97 1 2 3 4 5 6 7 8 9 98 1 2 3 4 5 6 7 8 9 99 1	
	9 97 1 2 3 4 5 6 7 8 9 98 1 2 3 4 5 6 7 8 9 99 1	
	9 97 1 2 3 4 5 6 7 8 9 98 1 2 3 4 5 6 7 8 9 99 1	
	9 97 1 2 3 4 5 6 7 8 9 98 1 2 3 4 5 6 7 8 9 99 1	
	9 97 1 2 3 4 5 6 7 8 9 98 1 2 3 4 5 6 7 8 9 99 1	
	9 97 1 2 3 4 5 6 7 8 9 98 1 2 3 4 5 6 7 8 9 99 1	
	9 97 1 2 3 4 5 6 7 8 9 98 1 2 3 4 5 6 7 8 9 99 1	
	9 97 1 2 3 4 5 6 7 8 9 98 1 2 3 4 5 6 7 8 9 99 1	
	9 97 1 2 3 4 5 6 7 8 9 98 1 2 3 4 5 6 7 8 9 99 1	
	9 97 1 2 3 4 5 6 7 8 9 98 1 2 3 4 5 6 7 8 9 99 1	
	9 97 1 2 3 4 5 6 7 8 9 98 1 2 3 4 5 6 7 8 9 99 1	
	9 97 1 2 3 4 5 6 7 8 9 98 1 2 3 4 5 6 7 8 9 99 1	
	9 97 1 2 3 4 5 6 7 8 9 98 1 2 3 4 5 6 7 8 9 99 1	
	9 97 1 2 3 4 5 6 7 8 9 98 1 2 3 4 5 6 7 8 9 99 1	
	9 97 1 2 3 4 5 6 7 8 9 98 1 2 3 4 5 6 7 8 9 99 1	
	9 97 1 2 3 4 5 6 7 8 9 98 1 2 3 4 5 6 7 8 9 99 1	
	9 97 1 2 3 4 5 6 7 8 9 98 1 2 3 4 5 6 7 8 9 99 1	
	9 97 1 2 3 4 5 6 7 8 9 98 1 2 3 4 5 6 7 8 9 99 1	
	9 97 1 2 3 4 5 6 7 8 9 98 1 2 3 4 5 6 7 8 9 99 1	
	9 97 1 2 3 4 5 6 7 8 9 98 1 2 3 4 5 6 7 8 9 99 1	

97   98   99

Explanation. This cycle follows a temperature rise in the previous cycle. Thus, infertility lasts through Day 6. Mucus is noted on Day 7 and signals the onset of the fertile phase. The most fertile mucus ends on Day 12. Post-ovulatory infertility is determined according to the Roetzer mucus and temperature guideline.

1. Highest of the six lowest temperatures before the rise: 97.6°.
2. 0.4° above 97.6° is 98.0°.
3. All three temperatures after the cessation of the most fertile mucus type are rising and/or high temperatures.
4. The third high temperature after the cessation of the fertile-type mucus is at least 98.0°.

Infertility lasts from 8:00 P.M. on Day 15 through Day 6 of the following cycle. Thereafter, infertility continues according to the guidelines for menstrual/postmenstrual infertility.

Chart No. 13. (See page 172.)

Day 1: Menstruation (M) following a sustained temperature rise in previous cycle. 97.8°

Day 2: Menstruation. 97.7°

Day 3: Menstruation. 97.8°

Day 4: Menstruation. 97.6°

Day 5: Menstruation. 97.8°

Day 6: Dry. 98.0°

Day 7: Dry. 97.8°

Day 8: Dry. 97.8°

Day 9: Dry. 97.7°

Day 10: Dry. 97.4°

Day 11: Dry. 97.7°

Day 12: Dry. 97.6°

Day 13: Dry. 97.7°

Day 14: Dry. 97.4°

Day 15: Dry. 97.5°

Day 16: Cloudy mucus. 97.5°

Day 17: Translucent mucus. 97.3°

Day 18: Raw-egg-white mucus. 97.5°

Day 19: Raw-egg-white mucus. 97.3°

Day 20: Dry. 97.7°

Day 21: Dry. 98.2°

Day 22: Dry. 98.2°

Day 23: Dry. 98.3°

Day 24: Dry. 98.4°

Day 25: Dry. 98.3°

Day 26: Dry. 98.5°

Day 27: Dry. 98.5°

Day 28: Dry. 98.3°

Day 29: Dry. 98.4°

Day 30: Dry. 98.5°

Day 31: Dry. 98.4°

Day 32: Dry. 98.4°

Day 33: Dry. 98.3°

Day 34: Dry. 98.3°

Infertile: Day 1 through Day 15
Fertile: Day 16 through Day 21
Infertile: 8:00 P.M., Day 22

Chart No. 13

Date	Readings and Notes	
	9 97 1 2 3 4 5 6 7 8 9 98 1 2 3 4 5 6 7 8 9 99 1	
	9 97 1 2 3 4 5 6 7 8 9 98 1 2 3 4 5 6 7 8 9 99 1	
	9 97 1 2 3 4 5 6 7 8 9 98 1 2 3 4 5 6 7 8 9 99 1	
	9 97 1 2 3 4 5 6 7 8 9 98 1 2 3 4 5 6 7 8 9 99 1	
	9 97 1 2 3 4 5 6 7 8 9 98 1 2 3 4 5 6 7 8 9 99 1	
	9 97 1 2 3 4 5 6 7 8 9 98 1 2 3 4 5 6 7 8 9 99 1	
	9 97 1 2 3 4 5 6 7 8 9 98 1 2 3 4 5 6 7 8 9 99 1	
	9 97 1 2 3 4 5 6 7 8 9 98 1 2 3 4 5 6 7 8 9 99 1	
	9 97 1 2 3 4 5 6 7 8 9 98 1 2 3 4 5 6 7 8 9 99 1	
	9 97 1 2 3 4 5 6 7 8 9 98 1 2 3 4 5 6 7 8 9 99 1	
	9 97 1 2 3 4 5 6 7 8 9 98 1 2 3 4 5 6 7 8 9 99 1	
	9 97 1 2 3 4 5 6 7 8 9 98 1 2 3 4 5 6 7 8 9 99 1	
	9 97 1 2 3 4 5 6 7 8 9 98 1 2 3 4 5 6 7 8 9 99 1	
	9 97 1 2 3 4 5 6 7 8 9 98 1 2 3 4 5 6 7 8 9 99 1	
	9 97 1 2 3 4 5 6 7 8 9 98 1 2 3 4 5 6 7 8 9 99 1	
	9 97 1 2 3 4 5 6 7 8 9 98 1 2 3 4 5 6 7 8 9 99 1	
	9 97 1 2 3 4 5 6 7 8 9 98 1 2 3 4 5 6 7 8 9 99 1	
	9 97 1 2 3 4 5 6 7 8 9 98 1 2 3 4 5 6 7 8 9 99 1	
	9 97 1 2 3 4 5 6 7 8 9 98 1 2 3 4 5 6 7 8 9 99 1	
	9 97 1 2 3 4 5 6 7 8 9 98 1 2 3 4 5 6 7 8 9 99 1	
	9 97 1 2 3 4 5 6 7 8 9 98 1 2 3 4 5 6 7 8 9 99 1	
	9 97 1 2 3 4 5 6 7 8 9 98 1 2 3 4 5 6 7 8 9 99 1	
	9 97 1 2 3 4 5 6 7 8 9 98 1 2 3 4 5 6 7 8 9 99 1	
	9 97 1 2 3 4 5 6 7 8 9 98 1 2 3 4 5 6 7 8 9 99 1	
	9 97 1 2 3 4 5 6 7 8 9 98 1 2 3 4 5 6 7 8 9 99 1	
	9 97 1 2 3 4 5 6 7 8 9 98 1 2 3 4 5 6 7 8 9 99 1	
	9 97 1 2 3 4 5 6 7 8 9 98 1 2 3 4 5 6 7 8 9 99 1	
	9 97 1 2 3 4 5 6 7 8 9 98 1 2 3 4 5 6 7 8 9 99 1	
	9 97 1 2 3 4 5 6 7 8 9 98 1 2 3 4 5 6 7 8 9 99 1	
	9 97 1 2 3 4 5 6 7 8 9 98 1 2 3 4 5 6 7 8 9 99 1	
	9 97 1 2 3 4 5 6 7 8 9 98 1 2 3 4 5 6 7 8 9 99 1	
	9 97 1 2 3 4 5 6 7 8 9 98 1 2 3 4 5 6 7 8 9 99 1	
	9 97 1 2 3 4 5 6 7 8 9 98 1 2 3 4 5 6 7 8 9 99 1	
	9 97 1 2 3 4 5 6 7 8 9 98 1 2 3 4 5 6 7 8 9 99 1	
	9 97 1 2 3 4 5 6 7 8 9 98 1 2 3 4 5 6 7 8 9 99 1	
	9 97 1 2 3 4 5 6 7 8 9 98 1 2 3 4 5 6 7 8 9 99 1	

97   98   99

Chart No. 14. (See page 174.)

Day 1: Menstruation fol-
         lowing sustained
         temperature rise
         in previous
         cycle. 98.6°
Day 2: Menstruation.
         98.1°
Day 3: Menstruation.
         97.7°
Day 4: Menstruation.
         98.0°
Day 5: Menstruation.
         97.8°
Day 6: Dry. 97.4°
Day 7: Dry. 97.2°
Day 8: Dry. 97.5°
Day 9: Wet sensation.
         97.6°
Day 10: Tacky, yellow
         mucus. 97.3°
Day 11: Tacky, yellow
         mucus. 97.3°
Day 12: Tacky, yellow
         mucus. 97.3°

Day 13: Slippery sensa-
         tion. 97.4°
Day 14: Slippery sensa-
         tion. 97.6°
Day 15: Slippery sensa-
         tion. 97.8°
Day 16: Slippery sensa-
         tion. 97.5°
Day 17: Raw-egg-white
         mucus. 98.1°
Day 18: Raw-egg-white
         mucus. 97.9°
Day 19: Dry. 98.0°
Day 20: Dry. 98.1°
Day 21: Dry. 98.0°
Day 22: Dry. 98.0°
Day 23: Dry. 98.0°
Day 24: Dry. 98.0°
Day 25: Dry. 98.0°
Day 26: Dry. 97.8°
Day 27: Dry. 98.0°

Infertile: Through Day 8
Fertile: Day 9 through Day 20
Infertile: 8:00 P.M., Day 21

Chart No. 14

Date	Readings and Notes
	9 97 1 2 3 4 5 6 7 8 9 98 1 2 3 4 5 6 7 8 9 99 1
	9 97 1 2 3 4 5 6 7 8 9 98 1 2 3 4 5 6 7 8 9 99 1
	9 97 1 2 3 4 5 6 7 8 9 98 1 2 3 4 5 6 7 8 9 99 1
	9 97 1 2 3 4 5 6 7 8 9 98 1 2 3 4 5 6 7 8 9 99 1
	9 97 1 2 3 4 5 6 7 8 9 98 1 2 3 4 5 6 7 8 9 99 1
	9 97 1 2 3 4 5 6 7 8 9 98 1 2 3 4 5 6 7 8 9 99 1
	9 97 1 2 3 4 5 6 7 8 9 98 1 2 3 4 5 6 7 8 9 99 1
	9 97 1 2 3 4 5 6 7 8 9 98 1 2 3 4 5 6 7 8 9 99 1
	9 97 1 2 3 4 5 6 7 8 9 98 1 2 3 4 5 6 7 8 9 99 1
	9 97 1 2 3 4 5 6 7 8 9 98 1 2 3 4 5 6 7 8 9 99 1
	9 97 1 2 3 4 5 6 7 8 9 98 1 2 3 4 5 6 7 8 9 99 1
	9 97 1 2 3 4 5 6 7 8 9 98 1 2 3 4 5 6 7 8 9 99 1
	9 97 1 2 3 4 5 6 7 8 9 98 1 2 3 4 5 6 7 8 9 99 1
	9 97 1 2 3 4 5 6 7 8 9 98 1 2 3 4 5 6 7 8 9 99 1
	9 97 1 2 3 4 5 6 7 8 9 98 1 2 3 4 5 6 7 8 9 99 1
	9 97 1 2 3 4 5 6 7 8 9 98 1 2 3 4 5 6 7 8 9 99 1
	9 97 1 2 3 4 5 6 7 8 9 98 1 2 3 4 5 6 7 8 9 99 1
	9 97 1 2 3 4 5 6 7 8 9 98 1 2 3 4 5 6 7 8 9 99 1
	9 97 1 2 3 4 5 6 7 8 9 98 1 2 3 4 5 6 7 8 9 99 1
	9 97 1 2 3 4 5 6 7 8 9 98 1 2 3 4 5 6 7 8 9 99 1
	9 97 1 2 3 4 5 6 7 8 9 98 1 2 3 4 5 6 7 8 9 99 1
	9 97 1 2 3 4 5 6 7 8 9 98 1 2 3 4 5 6 7 8 9 99 1
	9 97 1 2 3 4 5 6 7 8 9 98 1 2 3 4 5 6 7 8 9 99 1
	9 97 1 2 3 4 5 6 7 8 9 98 1 2 3 4 5 6 7 8 9 99 1
	9 97 1 2 3 4 5 6 7 8 9 98 1 2 3 4 5 6 7 8 9 99 1
	9 97 1 2 3 4 5 6 7 8 9 98 1 2 3 4 5 6 7 8 9 99 1
	9 97 1 2 3 4 5 6 7 8 9 98 1 2 3 4 5 6 7 8 9 99 1
	9 97 1 2 3 4 5 6 7 8 9 98 1 2 3 4 5 6 7 8 9 99 1
	9 97 1 2 3 4 5 6 7 8 9 98 1 2 3 4 5 6 7 8 9 99 1
	9 97 1 2 3 4 5 6 7 8 9 98 1 2 3 4 5 6 7 8 9 99 1
	9 97 1 2 3 4 5 6 7 8 9 98 1 2 3 4 5 6 7 8 9 99 1
	9 97 1 2 3 4 5 6 7 8 9 98 1 2 3 4 5 6 7 8 9 99 1
	9 97 1 2 3 4 5 6 7 8 9 98 1 2 3 4 5 6 7 8 9 99 1
	9 97 1 2 3 4 5 6 7 8 9 98 1 2 3 4 5 6 7 8 9 99 1
	9 97 1 2 3 4 5 6 7 8 9 98 1 2 3 4 5 6 7 8 9 99 1

97   98   99

Explanation. The couple is infertile through and including Day 8.

Fertility begins on Day 9, when the woman detects a sensation of wetness in the genital area. Mucus continues through and including Day 18, which is the mucus peak. The following day the woman is dry and the dryness continues through the rest of the cycle. Here's how the couple determines infertility according to the Roetzer guideline:

1. The couple cancels the temperature on Day 15 which is 97.8°. Thus, the highest of the six consecutive temperatures before the rise is 97.6°. (Review guidelines on page 158 for unusually high temperatures.)

2. 0.4° plus 97.6° is 98.0°.

3. The three temperatures after the cessation of the most fertile mucus are higher temperatures.

4. The third high temperature after the cessation of the fertile-type mucus is 98.0°, satisfying the requirement that the third temperature be at least 0.4° above the highest of the six lowest temperatures before the rise.

Infertility lasts from 8:00 P.M. on Day 21 and continues through Day 6 of the following cycle. Thereafter, infertility continues according to the guidelines for menstrual/post-menstrual infertility.

Some Final Words about Temperatures

By the time you have recorded two complete cycles on your own, you may be ready to reduce temperature taking to two weeks or less out of your cycle. To do this, you must take your waking temperature long enough to get six low temperatures to use as a base.

Cutting back on temperature taking. Many couples begin taking the waking temperature after the woman notices mucus. For example, if mucus is noticed anytime on Tuesday, temperature taking begins Wednesday morning.

Temperature taking continues until the third high waking temperature is recorded, provided it is 0.4° above the highest of the six lowest temperatures before the rise. If the third high waking temperature *doesn't* meet the "0.4° above" test, then waking temperatures must be taken on succeeding mornings until the requirement is satisfied. Temperature taking can then cease, to be resumed when the woman notices mucus in the *succeeding* cycle.

Short cycles. Waiting until mucus develops before you start taking the waking temperature can be a problem if you have cycles shorter than twenty-seven days. You may not be able to accumulate enough temperatures to establish the six lows. Solution? Begin taking your waking temperature the fourth or fifth day of the cycle.

Forgetting to take temperatures. It's very likely that you may, at times, forget to take your waking temperature. You may miss one day or even several days in a row. Don't be discouraged; missing a day (or a few) happens to everyone, and is considerably less of a problem than missing one or more contraceptive pills!

It's better not to omit temperatures, of course, but if you do omit one or two (or more), continue again as soon as possible. *However, try not to forget during your first six learning cycles.* In this initial period, be very careful to record all information about your fertility and infertility. If you're careful in the beginning, you'll gain enough experience to judge the approximate site of the low and high temperature phases from only a few readings. This experience will stand you in good stead if you later forget to take your temperature in a different cycle. However, observe this one cautionary guideline: *if you forget to take your temperature for a number of days, take a fourth temperature before considering yourselves infertile.*

For example, with experience you may notice that your low temperatures usually hover around 97.5° and 97.7°. In contrast, your high temperature phase is usually about 98.2° to 98.5°. If you unaccountably miss taking your temperature for a week but are sure that you've passed your mucus peak, begin temperature taking right away. If your thermometer registers 98.4°, 98.3°, 98.5°, and 98.4° on four successive days, you are infertile provided there are no disturbing factors that might cause a higher temperature reading.

Note: do not make this assumption concerning postovulatory infertility unless you have at least six cycles' experience with charting. You must have this experience before you can take short-cuts.

Charting for the Rest of Your Lives

In the first cycle you waited until you had observed a sustained high temperature before you considered yourselves to be absolutely infertile. In the second and third cycles you waited for two fertility indicators, mucus and temperature, to confirm the return of absolute infertility.

By monitoring mucus and temperature changes alone, you will have the security of knowing when you are fertile and when you are not fertile—*for the rest of your lives.* From now on you can be completely independent of anyone or any*thing* when you plan your family.

If you have also opted to examine your cervix each day, it's now time to learn a way to make an appropriate record. If you don't wish to learn about cervical charting, skip this section.

Reliability of the cervical sign. Before beginning, I want to stress that no effectiveness studies published to date indicate the reliability of the cervical sign. Some couples find the sign very helpful; others do not. If in doubt, follow the indications of mucus and temperature alone.

Learning the cervical changes. Recognizing the cervical changes requires no more internal self-inspection than you may have used when you checked your IUD string or the placement of your diaphragm if you used artificial birth control. If your hands are clean and your nails reasonably well-trimmed, you will not hurt yourself or cause any tearing or bleeding.

Check the cervix at approximately the same time each day. Many women like to check it in the morning; others prefer to check in the evening.

There is only one matter to bear in mind: check the cervix at a time *apart* from your regular bowel elimination. The reason for this is that a full bowel can distort the interpretation of the cervix as either "low," "rising," or "high." If you eliminate in the morning, check an hour or so later.

To make the cervical examination, stand with one foot on the floor and the other raised on the toilet seat, the edge of the bathtub, or on a stool. Push down on your stomach with one hand and insert the index and/or middle finger of the other hand up into the vagina. Pushing against the stomach with one hand helps lower the uterus a tiny bit so that you will be able to make contact with the cervix more readily.

If you use tampons, insert your finger in the same way. Aim your fingers in the general direction of your chin.

Shared interpretation. The cervix signs are objective but do require interpretation. For that reason it may be helpful to have your mate help you evaluate them.

It's usually easier for a husband to assist if you lie on

your back with your legs spread apart in a V. However, if your husband becomes the examiner, he must be the one to perform the "cervical check" each day of the cycle. This is not only for consistency of observation, but also because the horizontal position places the cervix in a slightly higher position. In contrast, when you are standing, gravity will lower it slightly.

There is another bonus to husband participation: it will give him an opportunity to observe your changing mucus secretions at the same time that he checks the position of the cervix.

If the vagina is too dry to accept his fingers, they should be wetted with water. Don't use anything other than water (such as K-Y jelly or another type of lubricant), because these substances will make it impossible to distinguish slippery mucus with certainty.

If water is necessary because of excessive dryness, this is probably an indication that the couple is infertile.

Best time to learn. It seems to take most couples up to three or four cycles—and sometimes longer—to learn how to recognize changes in the cervix. It might be easier to learn to detect those changes if you were careful to begin at a time when the cervix is bound to be low and firm and will feel resistant, like your nosetip. This time would, of course, begin a few days after the temperature rise and last through the menstrual period (which might be too messy to use for learning purposes) and the dry days thereafter.

As you enter the phase of combined fertility, the "nosetip" feel of the cervix will gradually change into the softer, more yielding liplike feel—and, of course, the cervix will be harder to reach. A cervix in this condition is another sign that ovulation is about to occur, is occurring, or has just occurred.

Correspondence to the mucus changes. As you become skilled in checking yourself for cervical changes, you will also see how closely they correspond with the mucus changes.

Here's how to keep a record of the changes.

Mark the chart with a down-pointed arrow (↓) when the cervix seems to be:

- Low
- Firm
- Of a consistency like your nosetip
- Descending again

Mark the chart with an up-pointed arrow (↑) when the cervix seems to be:

- Softening or soft, like your lips
- Rising
- High in the vagina
- Barely reachable
- Unreachable

If you also find it easy to notice how the os is opening, show it graphically. A tiny opening rates a smallish, tight little circle. But as the os opens farther day by day, the circle may be drawn progressively larger.

Problems. If you're not sure about the cervical changes, remember the "if in doubt, you're fertile" rule and apply it. If in doubt about the cervical movement, mark the chart with an up-pointed arrow (↑). If you can make a judgment about the os, draw an appropriate circle next to the arrow.

After you've marked your first chart, you will see that the arrows pointing upward and the bigger circles generally coincide with the developing mucus and the very beginning of the temperature rise. You will notice that down-pointed arrows and the smallest (or no) circles generally appear on the days when you're infertile.

Short-cut temperature taking. The following pages will introduce, for the first time, charts in which an *experienced* couple recorded temperatures for only part of the cycle. Again, this is something that you may decide to do after at least six cycles' charting experience.

Chart No. 15. (See page 182.) This chart shows the cervical changes and the other fertility indicators unfolding in a very nice pattern together. Notice that the mucus feels slippery (although in this case the woman didn't see it—just *felt* it), and at the same time the os is opened the widest and the cervix is high (nearly unreachable) in the vagina.

By Day 20 the cervix is low, the os closed, and the area is firm. This day is also the second day of the temperature rise and the third day after the cessation of the woman's most fertile mucus type.

The couple waits until Day 21 before considering themselves infertile because by that day they have *triple* confirmation of infertility (cessation of the most fertile mucus type, high temperature, and low, firm, closed cervix).

Chart No. 16. (See page 183.) This chart is an example of when the cervical sign can be most helpful. A continuous mucus discharge must be monitored carefully, since any fluctuation in the mucus type may indicate the onset of fertility. Generally, as long as the continuing mucus *doesn't* change and remains consistent (though constant) the couple can presume infertility. *However, this is a situation that is best dealt with under the guidance of an experienced teacher.*

Another matter: if there is any unpleasant odor or any unfamiliar discharge associated with a continuous mucus sign, you should be examined by a doctor to determine whether or not pathology exists. In this case, the woman had a healthy vaginal tract. This was a post-partum cycle; these often show a continuous discharge.

Chart No. 15

*A typical
mucus, cervix,
and tempera-
ture chart*

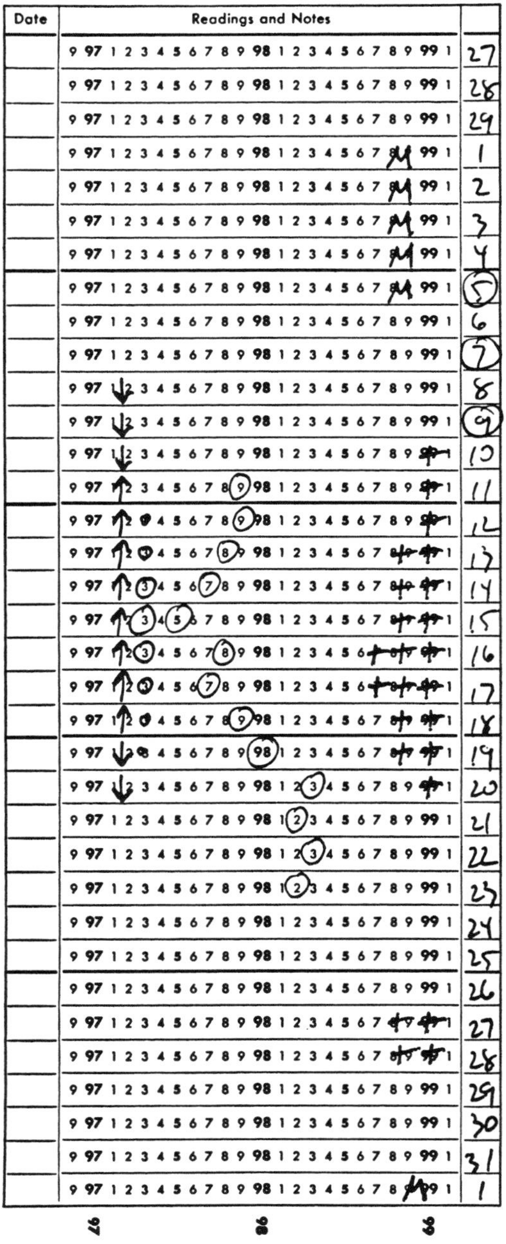

Chart No. 16

A continuous mucus discharge

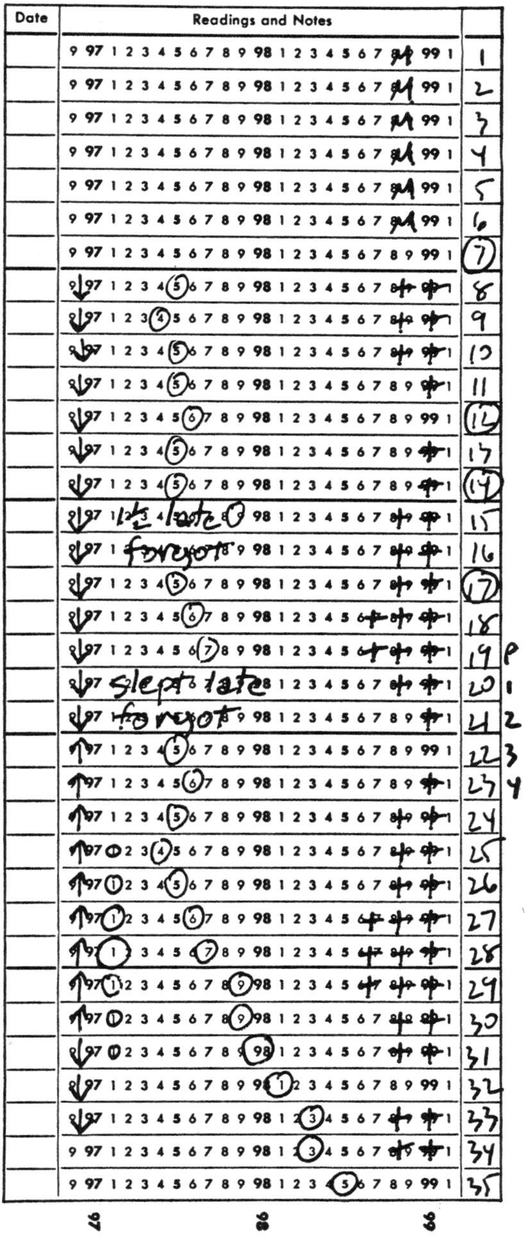

The woman is negligent about taking her waking temperature. (She sleeps late on two occasions and forgets on two others.) The temperature can tell her when ovulation has passed, but of course, it's of no use for indicating menstrual/post-menstrual infertility. This woman is experienced at observing the cervical changes. Thus, she discounts (though she records) information about mucus. You can see that the couple has intercourse when the mucus is of two-plus (++) quality because the cervix is low, firm, and hard. However, when the mucus changes to a more fertile type on Days 18 and 19, the couple considers themselves fertile even though the cervix is low, hard, and the os is closed.

Fertility. The couple observes the peak on Day 19 and considers themselves fertile from Day 18 (when slippery, three-plus mucus is felt) through the four days after Day 19. But when this count ends, the couple consider themselves still fertile for two reasons:

1. The temperature has not risen; and
2. The cervix seems to be softening and rising a bit on Days 22 and 23.

Fertility continues because:

1. On Day 24 and thereafter the mucus becomes more fertile; and
2. The cervix continues to rise and the cervical os itself is opening.

Infertility. The fertility indicators become more emphatic for the next several days. The most fertile mucus ends on Day 29; on Days 30 and 31 it reverts to a creamy consistency (++). The couple continues taking the waking temperature and by Day 32 they look back in order to:

1. Establish the six consecutive lowest temperatures just before the rise. (Days 23 through 28.)

2. Draw a line 0.4° higher than the highest of the six consecutive low temperatures (97.7°) before the rise. (Line is drawn along the 98.1° row.)
3. See if all three temperatures after the cessation of the most fertile mucus type are higher temperatures (i.e., above the highest of the six consecutive lows). They are.
4. See if the third high temperature is at least 0.4° above the highest of the six lowest temperatures just before the rise. It is.

The temperature and mucus signs indicate infertility on Day 32; the cervical signs also indicate infertility on that day. Menstruation begins twelve days later, confirming that ovulation may have occurred sometime between Days 26 and 29.

II

Special Situations

Although the fertility indicators we've discussed are highly reliable when used properly, various circumstances can affect your bodily functions, creating normal fluctuations in your usual rhythms and patterns. It's vitally important, especially in the absence of personal instruction, to understand these situations. You will then be able to interpret any altered fertility pattern that you may experience.

This chapter will cover:

- Coming off the Pill
- "Cycles" without an ovulation (anovulatory cycles)
- The post partum
- Miscarriage
- Effects of breast-feeding
- The pre-menopause

These special situations require extra attention and vigilance. Certainly there is nothing pathological or unnatural about them; they are merely different because your body is responding to circumstances that aren't present in your ordinary cycles. But *do* consult your doctor if you have unexplained bleeding, foul-smelling discharges, or any sign of irritation.

Coming Off the Pill

Women who have been on the Pill for any length of time before switching to natural methods sometimes develop a very keen appreciation of just how profound its physiological effects can be. Cycles may take a long time to return to normal, and in a small percentage of cases, ovulation may be delayed for months—or even years. A tiny handful of women are left permanently sterile because of permanent suppression of the ovarian function. Most women, however, experience normal cycles soon after discontinuation of the Pill. For some, even the first post-Pill cycle is normal.

Post-Pill pregnancy. Some health practitioners, researchers, and doctors are concerned that hormone residues from the Pill may be harmful to a developing prenatal child. *Thus, even if you wish to conceive, you are advised to avoid pregnancy for at least six months after discontinuing the Pill.*

Post-Pill infertility. Since the Pill's effects on your mucus may linger through several cycles, the mucus indicator should not be used to monitor infertility immediately after discontinuing the contraceptive. Furthermore, since it is critical that you avoid pregnancy during the first six months after discontinuing the Pill, the stringent guidelines you will be observing will insure that pregnancy does not occur.

These are the guidelines:

1. You are fertile from the day after you take your last Pill until the confirmed temperature rise according to the "6 and 4 and 3" guideline (page 121). After the temperature rise has been established, you are in-

fertile through the first *five* days of the succeeding cycle.

2. You are fertile again on Day 6 of the second cycle until you can prove infertility according to the "6 and 4 and 3" guideline. Thereafter, infertility continues through the *first five days* of the third cycle.

3. For six months after discontinuing the Pill, continue to consider yourselves infertile *only* from 8:00 P.M. on the evening that infertility is established according to the "6 and 4 and 3" guideline through *Day 5* of the succeeding cycle.

Observing mucus. Most women experience completely normalized cycles before the seventh month after discontinuing the Pill. But some women experience continuous mucus for days at a time. This is uncommon and hopefully won't happen to you. But if it does, just recognize that your body may have been more profoundly affected by the Pill and may take longer to normalize.

There is no need to consult a physician unless the mucus causes itching, swelling, irritation, or has an unpleasant odor. Beginning with the seventh month after discontinuing the Pill, you can chart mucus and follow the guidelines for infertility in the menstrual/post-menstrual phase found on page 143.

The cervical sign. You can begin trying to learn to recognize the cervical changes immediately upon discontinuing the Pill. However, most couples prefer to wait until the cycles normalize.

Chart No. 17. (See page 189.) This is from a woman who has been off the Pill for nearly eight months. She is still experiencing continuous mucus—an unusual situation. (Since the entire cycle would not fit on the chart, I arbitrarily cut out the first fifteen days, most of which showed mucus.)

The chart indicates the presence of mucus almost

Chart No. 17

*Post-Pill con-
tinuous mucus*

Date	Readings and Notes		
Jan 4	9 97 1 ②3 4 5 6 7 8 9 98 1 2 3 4 5 6 7 o⫿r o⫿�		15
5	9 97①2 3 4 5 6 7 8 9 98 1 2 3 4 5 6 7 o⫿r o⫿70		16
6	9 97 1②3 4 5 6 7 8 9 98 1 2 3 4 5 6 7 o⫿o o⫿70		17
7	9 97①2 3 4 5 6 7 8 9 98 1 2 3 4 5 6 7 o⫿r o⫿70		18
8	9 974 2 5 s *drinks* ①2 3 4 5 6 ⫿o⫿r o⫿r 1		19
9	9 97 1②3 4 5 6 7 8 9 98 1 2 3 4 5 6 ⫿o⫿r o⫿r 1		20	P
10	⑨97 1 2 3 4 5 6 7 8 9 98 1 2 3 4 5 6 7 8 9 o⫿r 1		21	1
11	9⑨7 1 2 3 4 5 6 7 8 9 98 1 2 3 4 5 6 7 o⫿r o⫿r 1		22	2
12	9 97①2 3 4 5 6 7 8 9 98 1 2 3 4 5 6 7 o⫿r o⫿r 1		23	3
13	9 97 *forgot* 7 8 9 98 1 2 3 4 5 6 7 o⫿r o⫿r 1		24	4
14	9 97 *forgot* 7 8 9 98 1 2 3 4 5 6 7 o⫿r o⫿r 1		25
15	9 974 5 *drinks* ①②3 4 5 6 7 o⫿r o⫿r 1		26
16	9 97①2 3 4 5 6 7 8 9 98 1 2 3 4 5 6 7 o⫿r o⫿r 1		27
17	⑨97 1 2 3 4 5 6 7 8 9 98 1 2 3 4 5 6 7 o⫿r o⫿r 1		28
18	9 97 1②3 4 5 6 7 8 9 98 1 2 3 4 5 6 7 8 9 99 1		29
19	9 97①2 3 4 5 6 7 8 9 98 1 2 3 4 5 o⫿r o⫿r o⫿r 1		30
20	9 97 1 2③4 5 6 7 8 9 98 1 2 3 4 5 6 ⫿o⫿r o⫿r 1		31
21	9 97 1 2 3④5 6 7 8 9 98 1 2 3 4 5 6 ⫿o⫿r o⫿r 1		32
22	9 97 *drinks* 9 98 1 2③4 5 6 ⫿o⫿r o⫿r 1		33	P
23	9 97 1 2 3 ⑤6 7 8 9 98 1 2 3 4 5 6 7 o⫿r o⫿r 1		34	1
24	9 97 1 2 3 4 5 6 7⑧9 98 1 2 3 4 5 6 7 o⫿r o⫿r 1		35	2
25	9 97 1 2 3 4 5 6 7⑧9 98 1 2 3 4 5 6 7 o⫿r o⫿r 1		㊱	3
26	9 97 1 2 3 4 5 6 7 8⑨98 1 2 3 4 5 6 7 8 9 99 1		㊲	4
27	9 97 1 2 3 4 5 6 7 8 9 98①2 3 4 5 6 7 8 9 99 1		38
28	9 97 1 2 3 4 5 6 7 8 9 98①2 3 4 5 6 7 8 9 99 1		㊴
29	9 97 1 *drinks* 9 98 1 2 3 ⑤6 7 8 9 99 1		40
30	9 97 1 2 3 4 5 6 7 8 9 98 1②3 4 5 6 7 8 9 99 1		41
31	9 97 1 2 3 4 5 6 7 8 9 98①2 3 4 5 6 7 8 9 99 1		42
Feb 1	9 97 1 2 3 4 5 6 7 8 9 98①2 3 4 5 6 7 8 9 99 1		43
2	9 97 1 2 3 4 5 6 7⑧9 98 1 2 3 4 5 6 7 8 9 99 1		44
3	9 97 1 2 3 4 5 6 7 8 9 98 ②3 4 5 6 7 8 9 99 1		45
4	9 97 *forgot* 8 9 98 1 2 3 4 5 6 7 8 9 99 1		46
5	9 974 5 *drinks* 1 2 3④5 6 7 8 9 99 1		47
6	9 97 1 2 3 4 5 6 7 8 9 98 1 2 3 4 5 6 7 8 M 9 1		1
7	9 97 1 2 3 4 5 6 7 8 9 98 1 2 3 4 5 6 7 8 M 9 1		2

every day until Day 37. Most of the time the mucus was creamy and somewhat translucent, as you can tell by the double plus (++) signs scattered throughout. Notice that on Days 19 and 20 the woman experienced a change in her secretions. She felt a sensation of lubrication in the genital area. On Day 21, when the mucus suddenly appeared tacky, the couple marked the previous day (Day 20) with a "P" indicating a peak and followed through with the four-day count.

But apparently the wife was not infertile.

The temperatures tell the tale here even though the couple has been very careless about taking and recording the waking temperatures. *It is imperative to watch temperatures carefully when one suspects high fertility in the offing.*

The woman does have one high temperature on Day 19—but look at the notation: "4–5 drinks." This high temperature must be disregarded. Also, if you look at the days following the mucus indicator that the woman *thought* may have been ovulatory, you can see that there is no temperature rise. The couple realized that they must continue to consider themselves fertile.

We observe a return to mucus that gives a lubricative sensation on Day 30. The three days following are also characterized by slippery, lubricative mucus.

By Day 34, the couple realizes that the previous day (Day 33) really *is* a peak. What's more, the temperature is up. However, this temperature must also be disregarded. See the notation for that day: "drinks."

On Days 34, 35, and 36 the waking temperatures are rising. The woman's most fertile type of mucus has also ceased. At this point the couple checks the lowest six temperatures before the rise, so that they can apply the Roetzer guideline.

1. Lowest six consecutive temperatures just before the rise—Days 27 through 32.
2. Highest of the six lowest consecutive temperatures —97.4°.
3. Three consecutive rising temperatures after the cessation of the most fertile type of mucus—Days 34, 35, and 36.
4. Third temperature at least 0.4° above the highest of the lows, i.e., 97.8° achieved on the day of the second and the third high temperature.

The couple is infertile by 8:00 P.M. on Day 36. Their intercourse (after thirty-six days of abstinence) is indicated by the circle around number 36.

The "M" indicates menstruation.

About abstinence. This couple's thirty-six days of abstinence is neither typical nor atypical of the post-Pill situation. This phase can be a trying time for both the man and the woman. Still, a long abstinence can also have its rewards.

Every NFP teaching couple has special memories of certain couples they've taught. One of these fondly remembered couples was a young post-Pill pair with a special story about abstinence. It was the worst story I had ever heard . . . and the best.

They were young—about eighteen and nineteen—and had been married about a year. She had been on the Pill the whole time, but something about it bothered her deeply. She said that she felt it was wrong to be using it, although neither of them held religious beliefs on the matter. Since it meant a lot to her to stop using an artificial method, her husband willingly agreed to learn a natural one.

They came to our class and everything seemed

to be going fine. Then they missed a session and we wondered if something were wrong. I called and the husband answered the phone. He was quite brusque. "No, there's nothing wrong, good-bye." That was the conversation.

I could tell something was wrong, so I asked my wife to reach his wife. She did . . . and sure enough, there were problems. It looked as though there might be a layoff and he'd be out of work . . . a drummer had moved in upstairs and practiced constantly . . . *and* they were in their third month of complete abstinence.

Naturally, we made an immediate appointment. They brought all their charts and the four of us sat down together. It took me about an hour to make sense of her notations, but I finally figured out where the couple had gone off the track on their charting. I was able to show them the days they could have had intercourse. Those months of abstinence would have been unnecessary if they had only called us!

The two were visibly relieved to learn that they had been mistaken in their charting and abstinence was coming to an end. I found myself apologizing that they had gone through such a rough time together. But she stopped me dead in midsentence. I'll never forget her words: "Don't! Don't apologize. The abstinence was hard, but I wouldn't have traded it for anything in this whole world. Nothing.

"When you get married, you don't really know how it's going to work out. You can't be sure if love will be there six months later, much less for good.

"But I'll tell you one thing that I now know without the slightest doubt: *I am loved.* And I also know that *we love each other.*

"These three months have been the most important of our lives. Because of them, we learned that we're in love for today—and for always."

"Cycle" Without Ovulation

An anovulatory cycle is one in which ovulation *doesn't* occur. Such cycles can occur at any time to anyone, although it is very rare statistically between ages twenty and forty.

Since there is no ovulation, there is no possibility of conceiving during such a cycle. Still, since there is no way to know that a cycle is to be anovulatory until *after* it has passed, you must remain alert to the mucus and cervical signs.

Determining infertility. You may notice that mucus will appear, then disappear for a while, and then reappear, almost as if your body were "trying" to ovulate. This "now you see it, now you don't" pattern is natural and often is found in an anovulatory cycle. Don't let it trouble you. However, consider yourselves fertile until four complete dry days have passed after the appearance of any mucus.

If you've incorporated the cervical exam into your fertility awareness experience, be sure to check it each day. If the cervix begins to soften, rise, or open, be alert to the possibility of a pending ovulation. Remember: there is no way of knowing *in advance* that the cycle will be anovulatory. *Always assume fertility when there is mucus unless you can prove otherwise.*

Temperatures and bleeding. Since there is no ovulation, there will be no temperature rise. However, there may be a bleeding episode, although it is likely to be light, since it won't be a true menstruation. (Remember: only a bleeding that *follows* a temperature rise is menstrual.) *Consider yourselves fertile during any bleeding episode* *that isn't preceded by a temperature rise.* Fertility continues for four complete dry days *after* the bleeding has ended.

After any bleeding episode, continue to watch for the possible onset of ovulation and keep to the menstrual/ post-menstrual guidelines.

Infertility. Infertility begins after the cessation of your most fertile mucus type, when you observe a definite temperature rise according to the Roetzer guideline (pages 51–53). If the temperature rises right after the cessation of a bleeding episode and is sustained, consider the last day of bleeding to be the peak even if you observe no mucus after the bleeding ends.

Once the temperature rise has been confirmed, you are infertile through the first six days of the succeeding cycle. Infertility continues thereafter according to the guidelines for menstrual/post-menstrual infertility found on page 143.

Chart No. 18. (See page 195.) Here's an example of an apparently anovulatory chart. On Day 11 the woman notices a slight amount of sticky, tacky mucus. The following day, Day 12, the mucus is creamy and milky $(++)$. On Day 13 the mucus is again tacky, so the couple assumes Day 12 may have been the peak. They mark the day with a P and begin the four-day count.

On Day 14 and 15 the mucus again becomes shiny and somewhat translucent. On Day 16 tacky mucus is again evident, so the couple realized that the *new* peak was Day 15. It's marked with a P and a new four-day count begins.

Also, notice the arrows for the cervix. On the twelfth day the cervix apparently gives the impression that it might be rising. It seems to be softening and rising for the following four days, although according to this chart, the cervical os doesn't open at all. Then suddenly on Day

Chart No. 18

An anovulatory cycle

Date	Readings and Notes	
5/4	9 97 1 2 3 4 5 6 7 8 9 98 1 2 3 4 5 6 7 8̶9̶ 99 1	29
5	9 97 1 2 3 4 5 6 7 8 9 98 1 2 3 4 5 6 7 8̶9̶ 99 1	⃝30
6	9 97 1 2 3 4 5 6 7 8 9 98 1 2 3 4 5 6 7 8 9 99 1	1
7	9 97 1 2 3 4 5 6 7 8 9 98 1 2 3 4 5 6 7 8 9 99 1	2
8	9 97 1 2 3 4 5 6 7 8 9 98 1 2 3 4 5 6 7 8 9 99 1	3
9	9 97 1 2 3 4 5 6 7 8 9 98 1 2 3 4 5 6 7 8 9 99 1	4
10	9 97 1 2 3 4 5 6 7 8 9 98 1 2 3 4 5 6 7 8 9 99 1	5
11	9 97 1 2 3 4 5 6 7 8 9 98 1 2 3 4 5 6 7 8 9 99 1	6
12	9 97 1 2 3 4 5 6 7 8 9 98 1 2 3 4 5 6 7 8 9 99 1	7
13	9 97 1 2 3 4 5 6 7 8 9 98 1 2 3 4 5 6 7 8 9 99 1	⃝8
14	9 97 1 2 3 4 5 6 7 8 9 98 1 2 3 4 5 6 7 8 9 99 1	⃝9
15	9 97 1 2 3 4 5 6 7 8 9 98 1 2 3 4 5 6 7 8 9 99 1	10
16	9 97 1 2 3 4 5 6 7 8 9 98 1 2 3 4 5 6 7 8 9 ⃝- 1	11
17	↑ 97 1 2 3 4 5 6 7 ⃝8 9 98 1 2 3 4 5 6 7 ⃝- ⃝- 1	12 P
18	↑ 97 1 2 3 4 5 6 ⃝7 8 9 98 1 2 3 4 5 6 7 8 9 ⃝- 1	13 I
19	↑ 97 1 2 3 4 5 ⃝6 7 8 9 98 1 2 3 4 5 6 7 ⃝- ⃝- 1	14
20	↑ 97 1 2 3 4 5 ⃝6 7 8 9 98 1 2 3 4 5 6 7 ⃝- ⃝- 1	15 P
21	↑ 97 1 2 3 ⃝5 6 7 8 9 98 1 2 3 4 5 6 7 8 9 99 1	16 I
22	↓ 97 1 2 3 ⃝4 5 6 7 8 9 98 1 2 3 4 5 6 7 8 9 99 1	17 2
23	9 97 1 2 3 4 5 6 ⃝7 8 9 98 1 2 3 4 5 6 7 8 9 99 1	18 3
24	9 97 1 2 3 4 5 6 ⃝7 8 9 98 1 2 3 4 5 6 7 8 9 99 1	19 4
25	9 97 1 2 3 4 5 ⃝7 8 9 98 1 2 3 4 5 6 7 8 9 99 1	20
26	9 97 1 2 3 4 5 ⃝6 7 8 9 98 1 2 3 4 5 6 7 8 9 99 1	⃝21
27	9 97 1 2 3 4 ⃝5 6 7 8 9 98 1 2 3 4 5 6 7 8 9 99 1	22
28	9 97 1 2 3 4 5 ⃝6 7 8 9 98 1 2 3 4 5 6 7 8 9 99 1	⃝23
29	9 97 1 2 3 ⃝4 5 6 7 8 9 98 1 2 3 4 5 6 7 8 9 99 1	24
30	⃝9 97 1 2 3 4 5 6 7 8 9 98 1 2 3 4 5 6 7 8 9 99 1	25
31	9 97 ⃝1 2 3 4 5 6 7 8 9 98 1 2 3 4 5 6 7 8 9 99 1	26
6/1	9 97 1 2 3 ⃝4 5 6 7 8 9 98 1 2 3 4 5 6 7 8 9 99 1	⃝27
2	9 97 1 2 3 ⃝4 5 6 7 8 9 98 1 2 3 4 5 6 7 8 9 99 1	28
3	9 97 1 2 3 4 5 ⃝6 7 8 9 98 1 2 3 4 5 6 7 8 9 99 1	29
4	9 97 1 2 3 4 ⃝5 6 7 8 9 98 1 2 3 4 5 6 7 8 9 99 1	⃝30
5	9 97 1 2 3 4 ⃝5 6 7 8 9 98 1 2 3 4 5 6 7 8 9 99 1	31
6	9 97 ⃝1 2 3 4 5 6 7 8 9 98 1 2 3 4 5 6 7 8̶9̶ 99 1	32
7	9 97 1 2 ⃝4 5 6 7 8 9 98 1 2 3 4 5 6 7 8̶9̶ 99 1	33

22 the arrow points down. The cervix is down low again; it feels firm and hard, too.

Can the couple be sure that ovulation *didn't* occur? For all practical purposes, they certainly can. Look at the temperatures.

Temperature taking began the day after the first mucus sign was noted, on Day 12. The couple kept looking for a temperature rise. It just didn't occur. They waited nearly a week after the last sign of mucus before having relations (Day 21). They kept an eagle eye on the fertility indicators, cervix and mucus. However, the woman stayed dry; the cervix remained low, firm, and closed tight. Thus, they continued to have relations. The "B1" signifies a bleeding. It was scant and was not considered to be a menstrual bleeding.

In this case (though you don't see it here) the scant bleeding continued through a third day. Of course, the couple didn't have relations, and afterward they watched carefully for indications of the onset of the ovulatory phase.

Though you don't see it here, the fertility signs unfolded as they usually do. There was an apparent ovulation followed by a genuine menstruation.

Miscarriage

Nature's solicitude is nowhere more evident than in the processes that unfold right after a miscarriage. Fertility usually returns immediately. It's almost as if nature wished to ease the pain of your loss by making conception immediately possible again.

If you wish to take advantage of peak fertility to plan a subsequent pregnancy, watch for the signs of fertility. It's also wise to begin temperature taking right away. However, don't be surprised if the readings seem high at first. After you conceived, progesterone entered your system to help sustain the pregnancy; after a miscarriage, progesterone levels may descend slowly. Wait a few days for the temperatures to lower and stabilize; they will.

If you wish to postpone conception after a miscarriage, it is best to establish a post-ovulatory temperature rise before resuming relations. Depending on how advanced you were in your pregnancy, there may be a bleeding after the miscarriage. This bleeding could confuse your normal fertility signs, especially the mucus. If your pregnancy was well advanced—say twenty weeks or longer —post-partum conditions could exist. In this case, follow the guidelines for post-childbirth fertility in the following pages.

Post-Childbirth Fertility

The return of fertility depends on whether you are bottle-feeding or breast-feeding. It also depends on whether or not you are planning to rely on natural child spacing.

If you are fully breast-feeding (i.e., no water or formula feedings), follow the guidelines in the section on breast-feeding in this chapter (page 199). Also, see chapter 12 for complete information on natural child spacing by breast-feeding.

If you have elected to bottle-feed or partially breast-feed (i.e., give water and/or some formula feedings), it is likely that fertility will return very quickly. But under all circumstances you can consider yourselves infertile for the first two weeks after childbirth. Thus, the conjugal relationship can be resumed anytime during this period, depending on the mother's health and comfort.

After the second week post-partum, charting should be resumed and the couple must assume fertility until they can prove otherwise. The mucus may be obscured by the lochia (post-birth bleeding and drainage), so temperature is the only sign that can be reliably charted.

It is not very likely that you will be fertile by the third or fourth week, but the possibility exists. A first post-partum ovulation has been detected as early as twenty-seven days after childbirth. However, ovulatory cycles as early as six weeks after childbirth are uncommon. It appears that if a bleeding occurs at about six weeks after the birth, it is unlikely to have been preceded by an ovulation. Thus, the bleeding is not even a true menstruation. In terms of specific figures, there is approximately a 95 percent chance that there *wasn't* any prior ovulation if bleeding occurs within forty-two days after childbirth.[1] For the mother who is fully breast-feeding, the chances are even smaller.

Still, during the post-partum phase, caution is your watchword and charting your beacon. *A couple with serious reasons to avoid another pregnancy must consider themselves fertile from Day 15 post-partum until they observe an unequivocal, sustained rise in the temperature according to the "6 and 4 and 3" guideline.*

Mucus and cervical signs. If you are *experienced* in using these signs, you may rely on them to determine your infertile days before your first post-partum ovulatory phase begins. Infertility begins at 8:00 P.M. on the *fourth* complete dry day after the cessation of any post-birth bleeding, draining, or discharge.

Once you have determined the first day of infertility, follow the same guidelines that you used to determine infertility during your menstrual/post-menstrual phases prior to your pregnancy. Especially remember that if you experience mucus on *any* day during this phase, you must consider yourselves fertile on *all* mucus days plus *four complete dry days* after the mucus has ceased.

Experienced couples are usually able to make use of the dry days and readily recognize the onset of the fertile-time mucus that announces the beginning of the first genuine post-partum fertile phase. Fertility continues until after the cessation of the most fertile mucus when the three post-peak high temperatures are recorded and evaluated according to the Roetzer guideline. (See pages 51–53.)

The return to your pre-pregnancy state. Many couples want to know how long it will take to return to their usual cycles. Unfortunately, a definite answer is not possible. Each woman is different. In fact, each pregnancy and its aftermath is usually different from every other pregnancy for the same individual. But in general, most couples experience the return of their usual fertility cycles gradually, usually within four, five, or six cycles, unless the mother is breast-feeding.

Breast-feeding

A special bond develops between mother and infant during breast-feeding, and nature seems to acknowledge its importance by assuring that this bond remain undisturbed by the demands of another baby for at least a year. In effect, breast-feeding acts as an ovulation suppressant triggered by the baby's suckling.

Chances for conception. In *The Infertile Period* Dr. John Marshall mentions a study in which 87 out of 1,227 mothers conceived during the year after childbirth. But of these women, only 2 were fully breast-feeding, that is, fulfilling 100 percent of the baby's liquid and food requirements from the breast. Six women were giving supplementary food and 79 were not breast-feeding at all.

But here is the interesting part: both of the patients who conceived while fully breast-feeding had experienced a bleeding episode once before conception. The conclusion to be drawn? Dr. Marshall believes that it is fair to say that the chances of a woman conceiving before a first bleeding episode when she is fully breast-feeding are small.[2] Dr. Marshall also cites another study in which the researcher found no instance of pregnancy among 500 lactating women during the first three months of breast-feeding.

Still, ovulation—and therefore the possibility of conception—certainly can occur and the chances increase the longer breast-feeding continues. So don't confuse breast-feeding with infertility—especially after any bleeding episode.

Return of fertility. If you are fully breast-feeding according to the definition in chapter 12 of this book, you will be offering your baby complete nourishment without the necessity of following a rigid feeding schedule. The infant will always have access to mother's breast, either for nourishment or just for the comfort that sucking offers both baby *and* mother.

This type of *full* breast-feeding (covered in detail in chapter 12) is the most effective ovulation suppressant of all: the baby's frequent suckling apparently stimulates the appropriate ovulation-inhibiting hormones. Thus, it is unlikely that fertility will return before the eighth or ninth week after the baby's birth. Even if there is bleeding anytime before then, it is not likely to be a *menstrual* bleeding preceded by an ovulation.

If you are *not* fully breast-feeding—using a bottle or even a pacifier partially or occasionally—you are as likely to experience a return to fertility as if you did not breast-feed at all. Thus, you should follow the guidelines on pages 197 to 199 in the post-childbirth fertility section of this chapter.

When to begin charting. If there is a bleeding episode, charting should begin immediately. If a bleeding does not occur, begin charting by the fifth week. This way you are most likely to detect an early ovulation.

The only sure sign of a recent ovulation, of course, is the temperature rise. But to be forewarned about the possible approach of ovulation, observe the mucus changes. You may experience a stretch of dry days interrupted by a day or more of either tacky, yellow, opaque mucus or slippery, lubricative mucus. Each time you see or feel mucus, wait for the peak and then follow with the four-day count before resuming relations. You are infertile by 8:00 P.M. the evening of the fourth complete dry day even in the absence of a temperature rise.

You are infertile on all dry days *except*, of course, the four days after peak. Be sure to consider the day following coitus fertile during the dry days. Thus, restrict intercourse to alternate nights on totally dry days. (See page 48.)

Any situation that results in decreased feeding (and therefore decreased suckling) may bring on ovulation. Watch for mucus and cervical changes at these times:

• Discontinuation of night feedings
• Introduction of milk as either supplementary or complementary food
• Introduction of water
• Introduction of solids
• Any alteration of the baby's feeding pattern because of sickness, irritability, or a change in the household routine (moving, holidays, etc.)

If ovulation has not yet occurred, it is practically guaranteed as the baby weans. Be especially alert to the fertility signs at that time. For complete security, consider yourselves fertile until the temperature rise has been established according to the Roetzer guidelines.

Pre-Menopause

At some point, usually between a woman's late forties and her mid-fifties, the ovaries stop responding to the follicle-stimulating hormone (FSH). This is the menopause, the cessation of the woman's reproductive activity. This phase in a woman's life is also known as the "change of life" and the "climacteric."

The end of a woman's reproductive decades rarely occurs overnight, of course. It's usually a gradual "closing down" that can last many, many months. It is a profound change both physiologically and emotionally, and the period preceding it—the pre-menopause—can be a very difficult time for many women.

Declining fertility problems. Since the pre-menopause can extend over a fairly long period of time, a woman's body adjusts gradually to declining fertility. This may be reflected in the random appearance and disappearance of mucus. Occasionally there may be a bleeding episode. Weeks or months may proceed without a temperature rise, marking a long period of infertility. On the other hand, the woman may suddenly experience signs of fertility for months at a time. The pre-menopause is, indeed, a difficult, confusing time.

One fact helps to ease the minds of most couples going through the pre-menopause: fertility is greatly reduced during the "change." There are two reasons for this:

1. Some cycles will be anovulatory, making conception impossible anytime during the cycle.
2. When an ovulation does occur, the time between the egg's release and the following menstruation may be shortened to less than the average two weeks. As a result, a possible pregnancy may be unable to continue, since the uterine lining will be shed by menstruation before implantation can take place.

Temperature. Temperature taking at this time will offer you special security. With a daily reading you can be confident that ovulation has *not* taken place even if you haven't menstruated for a long time. If the temperature remains at a high level more than nineteen days following the ovulatory phase, you are very likely pregnant. (See page 45.) But don't forget: statistically, pregnancy is rare.

Menstruation. You may experience bleeding and occasional spotting during the pre-menopause. *Consider yourselves fertile during any bleeding episode unless it follows a sustained temperature rise.* Again, the only sure way to know about a probable ovulation is by taking your waking temperature and noting the sustained temperature rise.

If you are concerned about bleeding, or if it increases in quantity or incidence, have a doctor examine you.

If you've neglected temperature taking around the time of a bleeding episode and aren't sure you're infertile, wait until four full dry days have passed after the bleeding before considering yourselves infertile.

Pre-menopause guidelines. Because of the special conditions surrounding the pre-menopause, the guidelines for infertility are modified a bit:

1. You are infertile according to the Roetzer guideline (pages 51–53) through *only* the first three or four days of a new cycle. Thus, you may not rely on infertility through Day 6 and you may not be able to use the 21-day rule. The reason for these restrictions is that unusually short cycles with early ovulations are not uncommon during the pre-menopause.

2. You are infertile during all dry days if they are not part of a four-day count after a mucus patch.

Pre-menopause mucus. Dryness tends to prevail for most women during the pre-menopause. Thus, a couple can express their love coitally throughout most of the pre-menopause without conception occurring.

Some women, however, experience continuous mucus that fits the one plus (+) description category (see page

138). This may make it more difficult to evaluate infertility. Observe these guidelines for continuous mucus:

1. If you are familiar with, and confident in, the cervical sign, you may use it to determine infertility. But if in doubt, you're fertile!
2. If you are not familiar with the cervical sign, wait out the mucus for one or two cycles. After that, you may begin to consider yourselves infertile during the days of continuous one-plus (+) mucus if you feel you are able to detect a change to a more fertile two-plus (++) mucus *at least five days* before your peak sign.

There is one exception to this: you are fertile on days that follow an act of intercourse the previous night or in the morning. This is to insure that there is no confusion of seminal residues with changing mucus.

3. Consider yourselves fertile during all episodes of two-plus (++) or three-plus (+++) mucus. Remember that fertility continues for four full days past any appearance of such mucus. Infertility resumes after 8:00 P.M on the evening of the fourth day.

Hot flashes. A typical hot flash occurs suddenly. It affects the upper part of your body, causing the skin to redden, get heated, and sweat. Usually the flash disappears within minutes, although you may experience a number of them throughout a single day and night. The flashes may continue over a period of weeks, disappear for a few weeks, and return.

However annoying, hot flashes have a benefit: any day or days that you experience hot flashes, your estrogen levels are too low to bring on ovulation. These days may be considered infertile provided, of course, you are *not* experiencing fertile-time mucus.

III

Fertility Awareness:
Unexpected Benefits

12

How to Space Your Children Naturally by Breast-Feeding

More and more couples are developing a special love-style that involves no abstinence during the early years of married life: natural child spacing through breast-feeding. This particular approach is especially recommended by Dr. Robert L. Jackson, professor emeritus at the University of Missouri.

At the 1978 Couple to Couple League convention, Dr. Jackson pointed out that it is desirable for most couples to have their children during the early years of married life. Noting in particular the nutritional advantages of breast-feeding, as well as its effect as an ovulation suppressant, Dr. Jackson recommends that a couple allow nature to space their children during their childbearing years.

There are many advantages to this approach. One is that a couple is free to have intercourse anytime during their early married life when sexual ardor is usually highest. After achieving desired family size, the pair can avoid pregnancy by learning and relying on the signs of infertility—an approach that Dr. Jackson highly recommends.

Other advantages of this approach touch the children of the marriage. For example, Dr. T. Berry Brazelton, a

Harvard pediatrician and knowledgeable researcher on infant development, points out that infants and children denied loving contact and communication for months or even weeks at a time risk growing up severely damaged. They may become emotional cripples, even retarded. With this in mind, it is interesting to note that an integral part of child nurturing involves an infant's need to suckle. In other words, breast-feeding meets emotional, psychological, and nutritional needs. Indeed, nature considers it so important that a mother be available to her child for the first year or two, that proper breast-feeding will actually signal her body to suspend ovulation for a period of time after the infant's birth. Result? A couple's children will be spaced approximately sixteen to twenty-eight months apart.

Breast-feeding to space the birth of children is so effective that a recent article in the *New England Journal of Medicine* stated that in the world at present breast-feeding "has a larger statistical effect on couple-years protection than currently available technologic contraceptive programs."[1]

The June, 1976, issue of the *International Planned Parenthood Federation Medical Bulletin* reported that "Lactation world-wide is estimated to prevent more births than all organized family planning programs and thus has a definite contraceptive action." This is another instance in which our technology fails to achieve essential ends as effectively, efficiently, and successfully as nature does.

In "Child-Spacing,"* a superb article that first appeared in *Child and Family*, Dr. Herbert Ratner demonstrates one compelling advantage of leaving the responsibility of spacing to nature: the difference in the number

---

* The article was reprinted in the spring, 1978, issue of the *International Review of Natural Family Planning* and reprints are available for $1.00 postpaid. Write: The Human Life Center, St. John's University, Collegeville, Minn. 56321.

of years you will spend with your pre-schoolers. If you space three children approximately four years apart, having your first when you are twenty-four, your second at age twenty-eight, and your third at thirty-two, you will be thirty-eight years old by the time your youngest begins first grade at age six. That means that you will have spent fourteen years with one or more of the pre-school set around twenty-four hours a day.

Now consider the difference if you space three children naturally: if your first child is born when you are twenty-four, your second when you're about twenty-six or so, and your third when you're more or less twenty-eight, you'll be about thirty-three or thirty-four at the close of the pre-school period—not thirty-eight. You will have spent only nine or ten years with kiddies underfoot—not fourteen.

If you have four children on this artificial four-year child-spacing regime, you'll be forty-two before the pre-school period ends; in contrast, you'll be about thirty-six with natural child spacing. With five children, the pre-school period is extended until you are forty-six with artificial spacing, and ends when you're only thirty-seven or thirty-eight with natural spacing.

Dr. Ratner enumerates some of the advantages of condensing the pre-school period:

> Nature's prescription not only shortens the obligations of the preschool period, (1) it brings youth to child-bearing and the arduous early child-rearing years, (2) it permits children to grow up with more intimately shared lives, (3) it closes the generation gap between parent and child, particularly valuable in the adolescent years, (4) it lengthens the joys of parenthood and grand-parenthood, (5) it allows for leeway in case of obstetrical misfortunes and tragic events, (6) it gives parents the opportunity

to reexamine their goals while reproductive options are still available, and (7) it [permits the couple to] blissfully ignore birth control for nine years or more during the period of greatest sexual activity.

Natural ovulation suppression. Post-partum breast-feeding has several effects: it releases a special hormone called oxytocin that promotes uterine contractions, cutting down some of your post-birth bleeding; it also helps the uterus regain normal shape as a result of the hormones it maintains in the bloodstream. And, of course, breast-feeding suppresses ovulation. However, to bring about this last result, two conditions must be met:

1. Your baby must be nourished exclusively at your breast. Not even water should be offered; your milk is all the nourishment and fluid necessary.
2. Nursing should be frequent throughout the day and night, all twenty-four hours.

Frequent, continuous nuzzling and suckling promotes the secretion of hormones that suppress ovulation, extending natural post-partum infertility for months. Instant, "empty the breast" feedings are ineffective: a letup or reduction in nursing may cause a cutback in the ovulation suppression hormone level. When this happens, ovulation is rarely far behind.

Health advantages. I have indicated that nothing is better for your baby nutritionally than your milk. Various studies have shown that in comparison to bottle-fed children, breast-feeders have:

• Between two and four times fewer incidents of respiratory infections;
• Between five and twenty times less diarrhea;
• Between ten and twenty-two times fewer miscellaneous infections.

Other problems that can plague newborns are remarkably reduced if a mother breast-feeds. For example, there is substantially less asthma and hay fever among breast-fed babies in comparison to bottle-fed infants. But by far the worst thing I ever read about the effects of artificial feeding was reported by Niles Newton in an excellent book entitled *Maternal Emotions:* "The risks of artificial feeding vary tremendously with the differences in environment. . . . When an attempt was made to introduce formula feeding among the village people of southern Egypt, almost every baby died despite the fact that vitamin supplements were given and presumably suitable formulas prescribed."[2]

Such a report is certainly extreme; I've never read or heard anything like it. However, the report was made in 1949 and formulas have come a long way since that time. Thanks to growing knowledge and information about the nutritional needs of newborns, formulas have improved drastically over the past thirty-odd years.

However, unknown factors will surely continue to be involved. At different times in the past, for example, bottle-fed infants have suffered convulsions; they've broken out in severe eczemas. The causes? At the time manufacturers didn't realize that the formulas were short of—and required—vitamins B_6 and E respectively. The problems disappeared once these important nutrients were added.

Are there other unknown advantages to breast-feeding? Of course, we can't be sure, but it seems very likely. That's why better health figures for breast-fed children will probably always prevail. Certainly there is a fundamental reason for such improved figures: a human mother's milk is *species specific* for a human infant. A cow's milk, of course, is specific for a calf and must be modified considerably to approach the success of human milk for a human newborn.

Drs. Derrick B. Jelliffe and E. F. Patrice Jelliffe point

out that new research reemphasizes the uniquely complex nature of human milk. Your milk is made up of over 100 ingredients in special proportions and in particular chemical composition forms that are unlike any other type of mammalian milk.

Dr. Paul A. Busam, speaking at the 1978 Couple to Couple League convention, pointed out that taurine, a nonprotein amino acid, is twice as abundant in human milk as in cow's milk. It is believed that taurine may be linked to brain development of the infant. Also, human milk is especially high in lactose and one of its products, galactose, a substance that is critical to the formation of one of the main constituents of the human brain. So it may prove that human milk is linked to brain power!

Effects in later life. The long-term effects of breast-feeding can extend through to adulthood, according to Dr. Robert L. Jackson. For example, the amount of cholesterol is higher in human milk than in cow's milk. This would seem to be a drawback—but apparently it isn't. "In animal experiments, it has been found that relatively high intakes of cholesterol are needed in early life to insure the development of appropriate enzyme systems, which are needed in later life to control the level of cholesterol in the blood," reports Dr. Jackson. There is evidence that this is also true for humans. An eight-year follow-up study showed that infants fed human milk had lower serum cholesterol levels than infants fed artificially. These findings point to a possibility that breast-fed babies may enjoy a reduction in coronary heart disease, even heart attacks, in later life.

Dr. Jackson also points out that formulas are often much sweeter than human milk. "This may habituate the child to an excessive intake of confectionary foods with cariogenic [i.e., tooth decay–causing] potential and to an increased tendency to obesity—the two major nutritional-dietary public health problems in our country," says Jackson. The doctor also points out that a growing body of evidence indicates that adult-onset diabetes may be a result of long-term obesity.

Of course, formula sweetness alone won't predispose a child to obesity if he or she becomes habituated to the taste of sugar. The composition of human milk changes as the baby suckles, and the fat content rises during the latter part of the feeding. Dr. Jackson believes this is an important factor in automatically developing the infant's appetite control mechanism, since fat helps the child feel satiated. In this way, the breast-fed baby learns self-regulation of food intake and may completely sidestep overweight problems in later life.

Thus, in many known and probably *unknown* ways, human milk is specifically designed to help your baby. In fact, each mother's milk is not only specific for a human infant, but is specific for her particular infant. For example, germs roost in every household in the world, but different strains can roost in different households. Your tailor-made milk will pass along immunities to protect your infant specifically against the germs in residence in your household.

Convenience. Despite all the health advantages, some mothers worry that breast-feeding is interruptive and inconvenient. Probably nothing can be further from the truth:

> I was prepared for a lot of bother, but I can't believe how easy it is to breast-feed. I remember buying formula, sterilizing bottles, making up the formula, getting up in the middle of cold nights to heat the bottles—not to mention sitting up in the living room feeding the baby. Ugh!
> With breast-feeding, the milk is always there, always sterile, and always at precisely the right temperature. Middle-of-the-night feedings are a snap: I

just place our baby to my breast and doze off. Now how can anyone consider that difficult?

Prolonged breast-feeding. I was surprised by how many mothers continue to breast-feed for years, literally years. One mother has been breast-feeding for nearly two and a half years. Is it inconvenient? Interruptive? Here's what she said:

> Our baby has become so much a part of my own rhythm that it's no more troublesome to nurse him than it is to have him in our family. It's soothing for both of us and never really interferes. If we're out shopping, we just wait until we get home. In fact, many times he has had to wait, but even at two and a half he understands that. I *like* prolonged breast-feeding. Nursing offers us a quiet, soothing time to share together.

Natural—Not Instinctive

Some mothers who begin breast-feeding for the first time think that something is wrong with them. They believe that their baby should automatically come to the breast, that they will automatically have plenty of milk, and that everything will work with automatic and marvelous precision.

Not so! You'll need a little guidance and some help when you nurse for the first time. Breast-feeding is *natural* in the sense that there's no interference from technology, but that doesn't necessarily mean it's *instinctive*. (And I'll mention that the same applies to natural family planning. It's natural—and not at all instinctive.) Unless you've been around breast-feeding mothers, you will certainly have your share of questions and will need some answers.

If I had to credit any one single place for answering

the questions of would-be breast-feeders, I'd unquestionably salute the La Leche League, an international organization with one goal: assisting mothers with the help, guidance, and information they need to breast-feed. Here's what one new mother told me—a typical story:

> I could never have learned how to breast-feed without the League. I had inverted nipples, plus my milk didn't come in for five full days. I was so worried and had so many questions that I called my chapter leader four and five times a day. I was that desperate.
>
> Imagine trying to call a doctor that often. You just wouldn't. And if your doctor were your only source for breast-feeding information, you wouldn't breast-feed either.

I urge you to contact the League for detailed *personal* help. They can also provide excellent books on the subject. See Appendix C for further information.

Learning to Breast-feed

Technology can inadvertently be a cause of some of your early learning-to-nurse problems. If drugs were administered to you during the delivery, your infant may be drugged for days after the birth, and may be too sleepy to suck properly—if at all—for the first few days. Result? *You* may think that *you* have a problem!

Certainly there will be a "problem," but it won't have anything to do with either you or your baby. You'll simply have to wait a few days to catch up completely on breast-feeding.

Milk quality. The early secretion from the human breast—colostrum—is yellow. When the real milk starts coming in, it may look blue. This is because the fat globules that give milk its characteristic creamy color are usually "caught" high in the milk ducts of the breast and don't descend when your newborn first begins sucking. Your baby's sucking will eventually bring down the fatty particles that are not only a necessary part of an infant's diet, but also involve the development of the appetite control mechanism. It sometimes takes ten minutes or longer before the milk looks creamy.

The "let down" reflex. Many mothers worry if their milk isn't immediately available for the baby. If you've never nursed before, it is perfectly natural if the milk doesn't come out freely at first. Don't worry about it. Your baby's sucking will eventually trigger the "let down" reflex, releasing the milk for the infant. Once this happens, the milk may come gushing out without any effort on anyone's part—yours or your baby's.

But remember: the milk may not let down right away —even for a few days or so—and if it takes awhile, relax. It's not abnormal and your baby won't starve.

Weight. If you're experiencing difficulties while nursing, and on top of that your infant is losing weight, you may worry that there's something wrong with your baby, with you, or with both of you. Again, there's no reason for concern.

Many newborns lose weight after birth, and the weight won't be regained immediately. It can take three weeks for your infant to reach his birth weight, whether he or she is breast-fed or bottle-fed.

Nursing frequency. For natural child spacing, breastfeeding must be continuous throughout the day and night. But what does that mean? Must your baby be carried around with you at the breast for twenty-four hours?

Of course not. Nurse your baby when he or she is hungry. It's as simple as that.

In the beginning, your infant may be hungry every two or three hours. Just put baby to your breast. Once full, he or she will probably go right back to sleep. Later, the hours of sleep between nursing sessions will lengthen. Don't worry about a particular schedule. The every-four-hours feeding schedule is a leftover from old hospital practices, when hospital nurseries had tight routines to streamline work. Let your newborn dictate the feeding schedule—not a mechanical clock.

At the beginning, you will probably want to nurse your infant at least five to ten minutes at each breast. As the baby gets older and stronger, the time that you nurse at each breast will also increase. Above all, allow your infant to snuggle and nuzzle at your breast. *You* should be your baby's pacifier as long as you're wanted.

Don't worry about your milk supply when the baby's nursing increases. You will have enough milk to satisfy the needs of one hungry baby, and even two if you have twins. A delicate harmony is involved in milk production. The more the baby sucks, the more your body will produce. But as your baby begins to wean himself (or if you deliberately begin weaning your infant), reduced suckling will signal your body to cut milk production. Your body always takes its cues *directly from your baby* to insure that there is enough milk available for his needs; neither too much, which would make your breasts feel achey, or too little, which would leave your baby hungry.

Sore nipples. If you have delicate skin, you may experience soreness from time to time. This is natural and shouldn't stop you from nursing. The soreness will generally disappear, particularly if you follow these steps:

- Keep nipples dry and exposed to air when possible.
- Never pull your baby off your nipple suddenly. Instead, break suction by pressing two or three fingers against your breast and pushing the flesh gently away from the baby's mouth.

- Vary your position when you nurse to distribute the stress and pressure evenly on your nipples.
- Avoid the use of soap or alcohol on your nipples. These substances are very drying and will only aggravate soreness. Use only plain water when you wash your breasts and nipples. Your skin's natural protective acid-mantle is antibacterial. You won't need to "disinfect" your nipples with alcohol or any other substance that may cause dryness.
- If your nipples become sore enough to need a soothing ointment, try ordinary solid vegetable shortening (e.g., Crisco). It spreads easily, is compatible with your skin's acid-mantle, has no dangerous additives, and won't harm your baby if he or she tastes it while nursing. This is *not* true of all medications and ointments that are sometimes prescribed, some of which must be removed before you begin to nurse.

It is rare for the nipples to become so sore that you simply can't put your baby to your breast. Even when you see blood, the nipples still are not so sore that the baby can't nurse. If you do see a little blood in baby's mouth, there's nothing to worry about. It won't hurt your infant.

Nursing with sore nipples. It is important to continue nursing if at all possible, but if you can't nurse more than seven to ten minutes on each side, don't worry about it. According to La Leche League research, an infant will receive about 90 percent of the milk within the breast within the first seven minutes or so of nursing. But the League stresses that all of his *sucking* needs—plus his need to be held and cuddled—can't be satisfied that quickly.

If you have serious problems with painful, sore nipples and must restrict nursing, you have a tailor-made opportunity to let daddy spend extra time cuddling and holding your baby. Infants don't go right back to sleep after feeding once they are a few weeks old, so use that interim to communicate love—by snuggling, holding, stroking, and cooing. The language of touch is totally, completely, and thoroughly clear to your baby from the beginning.

Milk expression. If you absolutely can't nurse because of soreness (a very rare situation, by the way), then you will have to squeeze the milk out of each breast yourself. This is called "expressing the milk." The milk must be removed; otherwise your breasts will become engorged and ache painfully.

Some mothers express a little milk before each nursing to encourage the "let down" reflex. This way the infant doesn't have to suck as long—which adds stress to the nipple—and there is less chance of soreness and cracking.

To express your milk, cup your breast in one hand, press the thumb and forefinger of your hand against the portion of the areola that is under the nipple. With the forefinger of your other hand, squeeze down on the part of the areola that is *above* the nipple, starting a bit to the side and then moving all around the circumference of the areola.

At the very beginning you may have a little difficulty squeezing milk out of the nipple. Don't worry about it; continue to try for three or four minutes. You may only get a few drops of milk, but that's still a beginning.

Switch to the other breast and repeat the same procedure. Again, don't get discouraged if no milk comes out at first; continue your squeezing for the same three to four minutes, then go back to the first breast and repeat. After that, return to the second breast.

Many mothers who work and must necessarily be away from their babies for a feeding leave enough of their own milk refrigerated at home so that the infant is assured of Triple A quality milk. If you want to do this, express the milk right into a clean cup and transfer it to a bottle. Many mothers freeze their milk so that the baby can have breast milk if mother has to be away even longer. And, yes, breast milk *can* be frozen. However, don't keep your milk in the freezer longer than two weeks. If an opportunity to use it hasn't arrived by that time, discard it.

Breast infection. Occasionally a woman can develop a breast infection, or even a breast abscess, while nursing. If it happens to you, please don't get too worried—and *don't* cut back on breast-feeding.

In *Nursing Your Baby*—a book that I highly recommend—Karen Pryor describes an experiment conducted by Dr. E. Robbins Kimball of Northwestern University Medical School. He had two groups of women who developed breast infections. The first group of 100 women were given antibiotics and told to nurse very frequently to keep their breasts empty. All signs of infection disappeared for these women within a few days.

The second group—only thirty women—received antibiotics but weaned their infants immediately. According to Pryor: "All thirty developed abscesses, fifteen required surgery, and none recovered in less than sixty days."[3]

Another problem that can sometimes develop is the so-called "caked" breast in which one or two ducts become blocked temporarily by milk secretions. You may notice a soreness and redness; a low-grade fever may even develop. Again, proper treatment includes continuous breast-feeding. Here's what Dr. Richard M. Applebaum, a pediatrician with a great deal of experience with breast-feeding mothers, writes concerning such problems: "The physician should instruct the mother to nurse *twice as frequently* on the affected breast. *Above all, he must not tell the mother to stop nursing!*"[4] (Emphasis is Applebaum's.)

The caking and lumpiness can be uncomfortable. Applebaum recommends continuous application of hot, wet compresses and suggests that they be renewed hourly.

He specifically mentions that a washcloth is preferable to a heavy hot water bottle. If there is pain, there is no reason not to seek some relief with analgesics. Check with your doctor for recommendations.

Weaning. When do you stop breast-feeding? Only one special person has the answer: your baby. Allow your infant to wean himself or herself over a period of months. If your six-month-old daughter sees food on the table that she wants to taste, let her. Of course, continue breast-feeding during this phase, allowing your infant to nurse without restrictions. Remember: nursing handles a multitude of important functions, and one of them is giving your child *you*—your warmth, your touch, your fondling, your cooing. It's your first important sustained child-nurturing activity.

13

How to Overcome Infertility Problems

Of the many benefits of natural family planning, one is unheralded: it is the only family planning method that works "in reverse" to help you achieve pregnancy. Here are three case histories:

Case #1: This couple had been unable to achieve pregnancy for nearly two years. They learned why with fertility awareness. Unwittingly, the couple had never had relations during their fertile phase because the wife felt achey and bloated around the time of ovulation—*her* individual fertility sign. The couple conceived during their first cycle of charting.

Case #2: A couple was unable to conceive for several years after "trying very hard." Upon questioning, the doctor learned that the couple was trying very hard indeed: they had relations every day of the cycle except the days of menstruation. The doctor suspected that such frequency of intercourse was keeping the sperm count too low to achieve conception.

The woman was taught to observe the changes in her cervical mucus secretions. The couple began abstinence to build the supply of fresh, viable sperm. Abstinence ended the day the woman noticed the slippery sensation of raw-egg-white mucus in the genital area. The couple conceived in the first cycle.

Case #3: A couple trying to achieve pregnancy were frequently separated because of the husband's traveling job. Once the couple learned fertility awareness, they recognized that the optimum time for conception was going to occur during a time when the husband would be out of town. Solution? The two children were sent to Grannie's for a four-day visit while the wife went on the business trip. The couple didn't conceive on the first trip, but they did on the second.

Infertility on the rise. With so many articles and books written about avoiding pregnancy, it's easy to forget that there is a growing minority with a different problem: they want to get pregnant and can't. As a matter of record, experts agree that the problem of infertility is a growing one. Today it is estimated that as many as one out of eight or nine couples are having difficulty achieving a desired pregnancy.

Why is infertility more of a problem today than in the past? There are several reasons; three are relevant here.

1. Use of the Pill. Sometimes the ovulation suppression action of the Pill persists after discontinuation. Ovulation usually returns spontaneously, but there are cases in which suppression is apparently permanent, even after use of fertility drugs.

Some women are not infertile after Pill discontinuation, but are unable to carry a pregnancy to term, since every one spontaneously aborts. The miscarriages may or may not be a result of having taken the Pill.

2. Use of the IUD. Pelvic infections are not uncommon and can damage the Fallopian tubes, making conception difficult or impossible. The damage can be corrected in some cases, not in others. One infection was so severe that both tubes had to be surgically removed, rendering a young wife in her early twenties with no children permanently sterile. At this writing the couple is considering a lawsuit against the IUD manufacturer.

3. Delaying childbearing. Chances for conception within six months is about 80 percent for random attempts if the wife is in her early twenties; 35 to 40 percent if she waits until her early thirties. (There are no figures available for the couple who can accurately bracket the fertile phase.)

Assuming there is no physical problem, a couple should be able to conceive fairly easily, since an average year usually offers at least eleven to fourteen ovulations—opportunities for conception. However, sometimes there are unforeseen difficulties. If this is the case and the couple has delayed having the first child, they don't even *learn* that there are complications until they are older, when the "youth advantage" is irretrievably lost.

Planning ahead. Many infertility experts urge couples not to delay childbearing, to ask themselves, "How old will we be when our last child is born?" It is preferable if the wife is in her early thirties when the last child is born rather than bearing her first child at that age. Remember: there is only one day in your cycle when you can possibly conceive, so you have an average of approximately eleven to fourteen opportunities in one year to achieve conception, depending on the length of your cycles. If childbearing is delayed, it is possible that all the opportunities to conceive within one year will be expended before you even begin to realize that you have a problem.

Once you recognize that there is a difficulty and begin your visits to a doctor who might be able to help, additional opportunities to conceive—at least one and very likely two or three—will pass as the physician tries to assess the problem. Meanwhile, you are growing older, and your options are narrowing apace.

Fertility awareness and infertility. Three questionnaires came from people coping with the sorrow of an infertility problem—a couple responding together and a wife responding alone. One of the wives, age forty-one, is a registered nurse. I thought her comments were remarkable because of her medical background and training:

> I have tried for years to achieve a pregnancy. Our boy is adopted. I'm weary of seeking help through gynecologists; it's expensive, sometimes humiliating, and it's depressing never to achieve.
>
> Although I was seen at an infertility clinic at a university hospital and have been on fertility drugs for years, *no one* taught me what NFP did. I feel that if I had only been taught this—how to tell when I ovulate—maybe I would have achieved that wanted pregnancy. Because my husband's sperm count is low, but supposedly adequate, and because I was on fertility drugs, timing was all important. But we never knew on which day I ovulated. NFP has an important story to tell.

It is not surprising that a health professional did not have ready information about the cervical mucus changes or the cervical sign. Many doctors don't fully recognize the meaning of these changes, and some physicians don't even recognize that they occur!

The second couple with the infertility problem talked about other problems:

> Going to a doctor to get pregnant has at least two drawbacks. He knows all about your fertility while you remain ignorant; and you inevitably become frustrated and broke because of the expense. NFP has no side effects and the couple gains confidence as they learn how to control reproduction.

Like the nurse and her husband, this second couple also had an adopted child and wanted to provide siblings for their daughter without adopting, "which today is a trying experience." But unlike the nurse, who had never used an IUD or taken the Pill, the couple's infertility problems were possibly related to the fact that the wife had been on the Pill for four years.

Even while she was on the Pill, the wife noted drawbacks. Her interest in sex decreased and her blood pressure went up. Still, the wife reported that the Pill was highly effective in preventing pregnancy, "but the methods employed were not explained to me or I would never have used it. The after-effects of the Pill have been so devastating that I would certainly discourage its use."

After she discontinued the Pill, she began to discover problems:

> I couldn't menstruate for six months and had irregular periods for one year (eighteen months altogether). This is in spite of the fact that I had very regular periods and no problems whatsoever before the Pill. Now that I'm off the Pill, I miscarry whenever I get pregnant.

The persistent miscarriage problem—six since discontinuation of the Pill—is one of heartbreak and sorrow for a couple trying to achieve pregnancy. More than anything, the miscarriages are probably the "devastating" after-effects that the woman spoke of.

The woman also said that she found natural family planning highly satisfactory, since it had directly helped the couple to achieve two of the six desired pregnancies. "Even though I miscarried later, up to then the only hope I'd been given by doctors was fertility drugs. Now it happens that fertility stimulation was not at all what I needed, which makes drugs even more useless and undesirable."

Alternatives to drugs. Many women find that improving the level of their nutritional intake for at least six months to a year gives them a better chance of achieving a desired pregnancy. There is a reason for this: a healthy body is vital to reproductive normalcy. Indeed, long-time Pill takers often suffer nutritional deficiencies, since the contraceptive tends to deplete some of the body's nutrients. For a short list of recommended reading in this area, please check Appendix D.

What NFP Can Tell the Infertile Couple

Statistically, about a third of all infertile couples are unable to conceive because the woman doesn't ovulate. A period of months spent eating nutritiously and taking supplements (especially the B-complex nutrients, vitamins C, D, E, and A, plus some of the minerals) may help stimulate ovulation again. This is particularly the case if an inability to ovulate is related to prior Pill use. It is now recognized that oral contraceptives deplete certain essential nutrients.

Of course, not all ovulation problems result from contraceptive usage or poor health. A pre-existing problem may prevent ovulation because of some unknown cause. If you have such a problem and are taking the Pill or using an IUD, *you are exposing yourself to birth control hazards that are completely unnecessary, since you can't conceive in the first place.* If you are using barrier methods, the contraceptives are unnecessarily interrupting every act of intercourse to "prevent" a conception that could never occur anyway.

Now consider the difference if you use fertility awareness methods. If you take your temperature every morning and discover no rise, you are alerted to a future problem relatively early in your marriage. What's more, you are alerted to this problem *while your youth is on your side.*

In contrast, couples with ovulatory difficulties who use artificial methods may not discover potential problems until at least a year or more *after* they have decided they want to achieve a pregnancy. Any number of years could pass—depending on how long they delay pregnancy—before they are abruptly made aware of the fact that they may not be able to conceive very readily.

Visiting a doctor. Fertility awareness will give you an advantage on your first visit to the doctor. Since ovulation is essential to conception, your doctor is going to want to find out if you are ovulating. Don't *tell* the doctor that you have been ovulating; *show* him that you have. Come for that first visit with your charts in hand.

If your doctor is satisfied with the evidence, he will be able to move more quickly to other tests to eliminate other possible causes of infertility. A likely test will involve analyzing your husband's semen. This analysis checks the volume of the ejaculate and the quality of the sperm—number, size, shape, and motility. A low sperm count doesn't mean that conception is impossible, but it does alert the couple to a possible cause of the problem. Sometimes a number of days of abstinence before your fertile phase will build up the sperm count sufficiently to make conception possible.

Infrequent ovulation. A few women ovulate only occasionally—possibly as little as two or three times annually and sometimes less. There may still be periodic bleeding, but remember, this phenomenon doesn't necessarily indicate that ovulation has occurred. It could be intermenstrual bleeding, which is not a true menstruation.

If you are relying on fertility awareness, you may notice that bleeding episodes do not occur after a temperature rise. The absence of the rise is your signal that you are not ovulating. This is important personal fertility information you should have early in your marriage while time is still on your side. You may then wish to reconsider pregnancy postponement, since your opportunities for conception are already limited and may decline further.

The condition of your Fallopian tubes. If your husband's sperm count is adequate—and you are ovulating normally—the doctor will probably then check out the condition of your Fallopian tubes to determine if there is a blockage of any sort. Tubal problems account for about another third of the infertility problems and some are correctable.

Your doctor will probably do a relatively simple test—slowly introducing carbon dioxide gas through the cervix. If at least one of the tubes is open, you will feel a sharp pain in the shoulder area when you sit up. Occasionally, the test itself will "blow out" small adhesions.

Male infertility. The cause of infertility could rest with your husband. A relatively common male infertility problem is *varicocele,* a varicose vein in the testicles. The condition is correctable with surgery and the pregnancy rate thereafter ranges between 40 and 60 percent and possibly higher if the fertile times are bracketed.

Sperm ducts could be obstructed, requiring reconstruction by a skilled surgeon working with special optical lenses to view the structures. There is a 30 to 40 percent chance of pregnancy after reconstruction.

The scrotum may be subjected to temperatures so high that spermatozoa are destroyed. Tight-fitting undergarments that keep the scrotum too close to the body may raise the temperature from body heat alone. Elimination of jockey shorts, jock straps, and the rubberized or plastic pants sometimes worn for jogging or running may restore fertility to normal levels within six to seven months or so.

The final advantage. Remember that the couple, *as a unit,* is fertile. As Lester B. Anderman, M.D., of Los Angeles points out, a couple's fertility is made up of the relative fertility potential of each partner. Thus, a wife with a high potential may compensate for a husband with a lower potential and vice versa. This means one thing: natural family planning can help some apparently infertile couples to *time* their acts of intercourse so that a conception is most likely to occur. The methods, per se, don't help the couple if there is a specific physical problem causing infertility.

Whether the problem can be corrected, is a matter of timing acts of intercourse, or is "just one of those things," fertility awareness adds a dimension of understanding. And if you become pregnant, you'll have 99 percent assurance of the fact within days of missing your menstrual period if your waking temperature remains elevated seven days beyond the norm for you. Then you can switch roles with your physician: give the doctor the good news!

Afterword

One question puzzled me during the hundreds of interviews that I conducted: how did the couples begin to use a natural method in the *first* place?

Answers ran the gamut. Typically, I was told that the method posed no health hazard to either partner. I was also told that it was more "ecological" and suitable to couples interested in a "natural" life style. A few couples cited the fact that natural family planning conformed to their moral and/or religious beliefs.

In fact, I knew that none of these reasons were sufficient. Calendar rhythm satisfies these requirements, yet almost all the couples had previously rejected that particular hazard-free, "natural," and non-objectionable birth control measure. Moreover, I recognized that virtually none of the couples interviewed would still be using natural family planning if they experienced surprise pregnancies. So I concluded that a critical requirement influencing the choice of any birth control method is that it be *reliable*.

But.even this brought up another question: why were the couples willing to give this new, essentially "untried and unproven" method a chance? Natural family planning is not well known in the United States. Its reliability is unpublicized, little recognized, and usually confused with the discouraging figures associated with calendar rhythm. Indeed, many women told me that their gynecologists derided their decision to rely on a natural method, assuring them that they would be back in their offices "soon" for pre-natal care.

So why, in the face of so little support, did couples risk a natural method? I often asked the question bluntly, but didn't receive satisfactory answers. Later I modified the question by asking why the couple hadn't opted for the diaphragm or the condom instead of NFP when they came off the Pill. That particular question struck most individuals as jarring. "It's not as nice" was a frequent response. "It's unromantic," "It's messy," were others. And, of course, "We did—and got pregnant" came up occasionally.

I concluded triumphantly that only two important indices were involved in a couple's choice of birth control: the method had to be simultaneously effective *and* free of interruption. I considered "proof" the fact that women were willing to tolerate such an incredible array of Pill symptoms *rather* than switch to a barrier method.

I also believed that Pill side-effects explained another reason why couples found natural family planning so satisfactory: selective abstinence can be difficult, but it's certainly more tolerable than many of the persistent physical side-effects suffered by many Pill users.* And, of course, the benefits of the method were considerable: high effectiveness without interruption of the sex act.

Today I realize that I was far off the mark.

My early conclusion reflected a rather "technological" view of human fertility. I completely overlooked an important, indeed a critical, aspect of human sexuality: the procreative function. Failure to recognize the importance of this function is tantamount to a failure to perceive an

---

* Curiously, few women in my sampling had used an IUD.

individual's humanity and personhood. I am particularly indebted to Dr. Ruth W. Lidz, clinical professor of psychiatry at Yale University School of Medicine, for valuable insights into this matter.[1]

Dr. Lidz reports that because the use of effective contraception involves the almost complete and certain frustration of a woman's procreative function, her general comfort, well-being, and self-esteem may be negatively influenced. It may also lead to a variety of symptoms, including depression.

Why such negative reactions? What causes them? Lidz notes several factors that may be involved.

One, of course, is the fact that fertility is a part of a woman's sexuality. This explains why virtually every woman is ambivalent about pregnancy at some time and some women are always ambivalent. Over the years a woman learns to adjust to this. Also, she can fantasize about a possible pregnancy if she uses less effective contraceptive measures (diaphragm, condom, and others).

In contrast, the effective artificial and surgical methods destroy that necessary ambivalence completely. Worse, pregnancy fantasies can no longer be sustained. In effect, a woman must adjust to the notion of sterility—a notion that is not congenial to many women and may negatively affect self-image and self-esteem.

Other studies indicate that the notion of fertility is very important to women. One group, studying the emotional adjustment of women who had been sterilized, found a striking correlation between successful adjustment and the presence of the unrealistic fantasy that pregnancy was still possible. Another study observed conscious pregnancy fantasies, symptoms, or signs in 152 women out of a series of 190 several months after sterilization.[2]

Today I realize that *whether it is conscious or not,* couples know that a natural method preserves the partners' sense of wholeness. This is because neither partner's fertility is suppressed in any way. And while a couple may choose to avoid pregnancy, they are not at the same time subverting either spouse's fertility. On the contrary: their joint fertility is not only recognized for the powerful force it is, but it also receives deference and respect from *both* husband and wife.

The woman receives particular benefits. One is that she can preserve that pregnancy ambivalence. She just has to remind herself—and women *do* remind themselves—that the couple can choose to achieve pregnancy at any time.

Dr. Lidz also points out that a conflict between wanting to be fertile and not wanting a child can be great. This is true, of course, and use of natural methods helps a woman realistically deal with her feelings and share them with her mate. Furthermore, natural methods prevent further emotional conflict caused by deliberate fertility suppression.

There is another fascinating aspect of natural family planning: use of natural methods requires both planning and a high degree of future-orientation from both husband and wife. This kind of future planning has helped some couples come to grips with their unconscious feelings that there was something "wrong" with sex. This fact was discovered when couples recognized that the idea of planning for intercourse was vaguely disturbing. Before, when intercourse "just happened," as it did, for example, when the woman was on the Pill, these individuals were able to "blame" sudden passions, spousal demands, whatever, for "what happened." Whether they recognized the fact or not, these individuals were not sexually liberated.

Once these couples changed to natural family planning and began to cope with the fact that intercourse had to be deferred *and planned for,* these individuals had to deal with deeper sexual feelings—negative ones—and begin the struggle to conquer them. But even more important, these individuals were *helped by their mates* to achieve sexual liberation. This is yet another example of how the communication and sharing fostered by natural methods can help overcome sexual problems. Once negative views were confronted, then coped with in a committed, loving, future-oriented relationship, these individuals were ultimately able to enjoy intercourse more than ever before in their lives. There is also a paradox: the apparent "restrictions" of the method played a key role in freeing many individuals from unconscious negative feelings about sex and sexuality.

Surely, natural family planning has many more positive advantages. These remain to be explored. At this writing, the methods are so new that little research or exploration has taken place, and there are still many questions.

Many individuals have told me that the change to NFP improved their self-esteem and at the same time deepened mutual respect. As one woman said, "I never realized how much my husband loved me until he threw away my Pills and made me go with him to our first class." Another woman said, "I never thought that Hal would be able to abstain for two days much less almost two weeks. I guess I didn't think much of him either."

In closing, I would like to share a well-known doctor's comment about the contraceptive Pill: "There has never been a drug that has been studied as intensively as the Pill." I suspect he is right.

I wish natural methods could get one-tenth as much scrutiny. In the long run it would probably be better for everybody. But it's not surprising that our university research centers and private laboratories are not expending this effort to study a natural birth control alternative.

After all, nature has no lobby.

Appendix A:
Personal Instruction in
Natural Family Planning

The Couple to Couple League is the largest teaching organization in the United States, with chapters in almost every state. CCL publishes a regular newsletter with the latest scientific information on NFP plus related subjects (breast-feeding, child nurturing, etc.). The CCL manual, *The Art of Natural Family Planning*, is considered authoritative by many in the field of NFP. For information, send a self-addressed, stamped envelope to:

> Couple to Couple League
> P.O. Box 11084
> Cincinnati, Ohio 45211
> Phone: (513) 661-7612

The Human Life Center will refer you to the teaching couple or teaching center nearest your home. Accompany request with a self-addressed, stamped envelope. (Note: a dollar donation to defray printing and secretarial expenses would be appreciated.)

> The Human Life Center
> St. John's University
> Collegeville, Minn. 56321

The following organization funds research in natural family planning and makes referrals to teaching organizations. Send a self-addressed, stamped envelope to:

Human Life and Natural Family Planning Foundation
1511 "K" Street, N.W.
Suite 305
Washington, D.C. 20005

Carman and Jean Fallace, consultants for this book, are founders of Family Life Promotion of New York. For information and referrals, send a self-addressed, stamped envelope to:

Family Life Promotion
P.O. Box 489
Smithtown, N.Y. 11787
Phone: (516) 929-6044

One of the best-known Canadian teaching organizations is Serena. For information, write:

SERENA Canada
55 Parkdale
Ottawa, Ontario, K1Y 1E5
Canada
Phone: (613) 728-6536

Appendix B: Charts

The charts used in this book were created by Linacre Laboratories, makers of the Ovulindex (BBT) thermometer. But if you receive personal instruction in natural family planning, *use the charts provided by your instructors.* Use of instructor charts will give important uniformity that's essential for learners who want to ask questions about their fertility.

If you do not receive personal instruction and require more charts, order from:

> Linacre Laboratories
> Box 1938
> Grand Central Station
> New York, New York 10017

A two-year supply of full-size charts costs two dollars.

Appendix C:
Further Reading

For up-to-date research on natural family planning plus information on child nurturing (childbirth, breast-feeding, psychological effects of NFP, etc.) subscribe to the quarterly publication *The International Review of Natural Family Planning*. Annual subscription: $12 ($14 foreign). Payment must accompany order. Write:

> The Human Life Center
> St. John's University
> Collegeville, Minn. 56321

The Human Life Center also publishes a quarterly newsletter (with occasional special issues) giving current information on natural family planning, contraception, sterilization, etc. Annual subscription $6 ($7 foreign). Address above.

The Human Life Center book service offers a range of materials and books on NFP, marriage and family life, and related topics. Also included is Dr. Roetzer's own book on natural family planning translated from the German by Richard Huneger. Unfortunately, the book's English-language title has not been decided at this writing. Still, it can be obtained by requesting the Huneger translation of Roetzer's NFP book.

For a complete listing of other materials carried by the Center, send a self-addressed, stamped envelope (business size) requesting the complete list. Address above.

Child and Family magazine, published four times a year, carries articles on child rearing and nurturing, childbirth, natural child spacing, breast-feeding, NFP, marriage and family life, etc. Excellent publication. 1 year: $4; 2 years: $7; 3 years: $10. (Add $1 per order for all foreign subscriptions.)

Child and Family
Box 508
Oak Park, Ill. 60303

Natural child spacing and breast-feeding. All the books mentioned in chapter 12 ("How to Space Your Children Naturally by Breast-Feeding") are available from La Leche League. I particularly recommend Sheila Kippley's *Breast-Feeding and Natural Child Spacing*—the best treatment of the subject I've seen anywhere.

For information, send a self-addressed, stamped envelope to:

La Leche League International
9616 Minneapolis Avenue
Franklin Park, Ill. 60131

Appendix D: Further Reading on Nutrition

Barbara and Gideon Seaman's book, *Women and the Crisis in Sex Hormones,* offers advice on which nutritional supplements to take after discontinuing the Pill, as well as a chapter on "Vitamins and Minerals that All Women Need."

Any of Adelle Davis's books, including *Let's Eat Right to Keep Fit* and *Let's Have Healthy Children,* offer valuable information. Dr. Roger Williams's book, *Nutrition Against Disease,* is a first-rate work that provides a fine understanding of how the internal biochemical environment of our body cells is linked with disease. Dr. Williams is a prominent biochemist who knows how to write without scholarly mumbo jumbo.

Nutritionist Dr. Carlton Fredericks's book, *Eating Right for You* is lively, even fun to read. It also gives you a load of solid nutritional information. Any of Dr. Fredericks's books are worth reading.

One can pick up nutritional information in easy-to-swallow doses by reading *Prevention,* a publication that calls itself "the magazine for better health." Send $7.85 for a one-year subscription to:

Prevention Magazine
33 East Minor Street
Emmaus, Pa. 18049

Notes

Chapter 2

1. H. P. Dunn, M.D., Oct. 23, 1977, personal communication to Paul Marx, O.S.B., Ph.D.
2. M. J. Muldoon, "Gynaecological Illness After Sterilization," *British Medical Journal,* January 8, 1972.
3. J. R. Neil, G. T. Hammond, A. D. Noble, L. Ruston, A. T. Letchworth, "Late Complications of Sterilization by Laparoscopy and Tubal Ligation," *The Lancet,* October 11, 1975.
4. James G. Tappan, "Kroener Tubal Ligation in Perspective," *American Journal of Obstetrics and Gynecology* 115 (April 15, 1973) : 1052–1057.
5. H. J. Roberts, "Voluntary Sterilization in the Male," *British Medical Journal,* August 7, 1968, p. 434. Also reprinted in *Vasectomy: Current Research in Male Sterilization* (New York: MSS Information Corp., 1973) , p. 119.
6. Andrew S. Ferber, Christopher Tietze, Sara Lewit, "Men with Vasectomies: A Study of Medical, Sexual, and Psychosocial Changes," *Psychosomatic Medicine* 29 (1967) : 354–366. Also reprinted in *Vasectomy: Current Research in Male Sterilization, op. cit.,* p. 102.
7. Valerie Beral, "Reproductive Mortality," *British Medical Journal,* September 15, 1979, p. 332.

Chapter 4

1. Gerhard K. Doering, *Proceedings of a Research Conference on Natural Family Planning,* W. A. Uricchio, ed. (Washing-

ton, D.C.: The Human Life Foundation, 1972), p. 172. Also, "Biology of Fertility Control by Periodic Abstinence," Report, WHO Scientific Group, World Health Organization Technical Report Series, No. 360, Geneva, 1967, p. 18.

2. Doering, *Proceedings*, pp. 175–176.

3. J. Marshall, *The Infertile Period* (Baltimore, Maryland: Helicon Press, 1967), p. 74.

4. Excerpta Medica International Congress Series No. 224, Advances in Planned Parenthood VI, Proceedings of the VIII Annual Meeting of the American Association of Planned Parenthood Physicians, Boston, Mass., April 9–10, 1970.

5. Josef Roetzer, *Fine Points of the Sympto-Thermic Method of Natural Family Planning*, No. 2 (Tokyo: Japan Human Life Foundation, Oct., 1977), p. 16.

6. Josef Roetzer and E. Keefe, *Fine Points of the Sympto-Thermic Method of Natural Family Planning* (Collegeville, Minn.: The Human Life Center, April, 1977), p. 4.

7. Josef Roetzer, "The Sympto-Thermal Method: Ten Years of Change," *Linacre Quarterly*, Vol. 45, No. 4 (Nov. 1978) : p. 370.

8. Edward F. Keefe, "Self-Observation of the Cervix to Distinguish Days of Possible Fertility," *Bulletin of the Sloane Hospital for Women*, 8, no. 4 (Dec. 1962) : 129–136. Also, Edward F. Keefe, "Cephalad Shift of the Cervix Uteri: Sign of the Fertile Time in Women," *International Review of Natural Family Planning* 1, no. 1 (Spring, 1977) : 55–60.

Chapter 5

1. William A. Uricchio and Mary Kay Williams, "The Mauritius Program," *Proceedings of a Research Conference on Natural Family Planning* (Washington, D.C.: The Human Life Center, 1973), p. 247.

2. Frank J. Rice, Claude A. Lanctôt, Consuelo Garcia-Devesa, "The Effectiveness of the Sympto-Thermal Method of Natural Family Planning: An International Study," paper presented June 23, 1977, at the scientific congress held in conjunction with the First General Assembly of the International Federation for Family Life Promotion, in Cali, Colombia, June 22–29, 1977.

3. John Marshall, M.D., and Beverley Rowe, M.A., "Psychologic Aspects of the Basal Body Temperature Method of Regulating Births," *Fertility and Sterility*, January, 1970, p. 17.

4. Charles H. Debrovner, M.D., "Medical, Psychological, and So-

cial Aspects of Contraceptive Choice," *Medical Aspects of Human Sexuality*, July, 1976, p. 33.
5. Peter Barglow, M.D., "Emotional Factors in Contraception," Ortho Panel, April, 1973, p. 17.
6. Ruth W. Lidz, M.D., "Psychological Factors in Contraceptive Failure," unpublished paper, pp. 9–10.
7. Charles V. Ford, M.D., "Psychological Factors Influencing the Choice of Contraceptive Method," *Medical Aspects of Human Sexuality*, January, 1978, p. 91.
8. Ruth W. Lidz, M.D., "Patient Motivation in Selection and Acceptance of Contraception," Mack Symposium, Wayne State University, Detroit, October, 1973. Also published in *Regulation of Human Fertility* (Detroit: Wayne State University Press, 1976).

Chapter 6

1. Viktor E. Frankl, *The Unheard Cry for Meaning* (New York: Simon and Schuster, 1978), pp. 39–40.
2. *The CCL News* 4, no. 5 (March–April, 1978) : 5.
3. Max Levin, M.D., "Sexual Fulfillment in the Couple Practicing Rhythm," *Child and Family* 8, no. 1 (Winter, 1969) : 10.

Chapter 7

1. Judith M. Bardwick, "Psychodynamics of Contraception with Particular Reference to Rhythm," *Proceedings of a Research Conference on Natural Family Planning* (Washington, D.C.: The Human Life Center, 1973), p. 197.
2. Donn Byrne, Ph.D., "A Pregnant Pause in the Sexual Revolution," *Psychology Today*, July, 1977, p. 68.
3. Mary Rosera Joyce, *How Can a Man and Woman Be Friends?* (Collegeville, Minn.: The Liturgical Press, 1977), p. 41.

Chapter 8

1. Iradj Siassi, M.D., "The Psychiatrist's Role in Family Planning," *American Journal of Psychiatry*, July, 1972, p. 52.
2. Bardwick, *op. cit.*, p. 212.
3. Cornelius B., Bakker, M.D., and Cameron Dightman, B.S., "Psychological Factors in Fertility Control," *Fertility and Sterility* 15, no. 5 (Sept.–Oct., 1964) : 566.

4. B. Kay Campbell and Dean C. Barnlund, "Communication Patterns and Problems of Pregnancy," *American Journal of Orthopsychiatry,* January, 1977, p. 135.
5. Bakker and Dightman, *op. cit.,* p. 566.
6. Barglow, *op. cit.,* p. 17.
7. Frankl, *op. cit.,* p. 81.
8. Abraham H. Maslow, *Religions, Values, and Peak-Experiences* (Columbus: Ohio State University Press, 1964), p. 105.
9. Ellen Frank, M.S., Carol Anderson, M.S.W., and Debra Rubinstein, M.S., "Frequency of Sexual Dysfunction in 'Normal' Couples," *New England Journal of Medicine* 299, no. 3 (Jan. 1978): 115.
10. Lee Rainwater, *And the Poor Get Children* (New York: Quadrangle Books, 1960), p. 96.

Chapter 10

1. John and Sheila Kippley, *The Art of Natural Family Planning* (The Couple to Couple League International, Inc., P.O. Box 11084, Cincinnati, OH 45211, 1977), Appendix 11, p. 206.
2. Josef Roetzer, "The Sympto-Thermal Method: Ten Years of Change," *Linacre Quarterly* 45, no. 4 (Nov. 1978): 369.

Chapter 11

1. John and Sheila Kippley. *op. cit.,* p. 133.
2. John Marshall, M.D., *The Infertile Period* (Baltimore: Helicon Press, Inc., 1967), pp. 77–78.

Chapter 12

1. D. B. Jelliffe and E. F. P. Jelliffe, "Breast Is Best: Modern Meanings," *New England Journal of Medicine,* Oct. 27, 1977, p. 913.
2. Niles Newton, *Maternal Emotion* (New York: Paul B. Hoeber, Inc., 1955), p. 52.
3. Karen Pryor, *Nursing Your Baby* (New York: Pocket Books, 1977), p. 97.
4. Richard M. Applebaum, "The Modern Management of Successful Breastfeeding," *Child and Family* Reprint Booklet Series, 1972, p. 41.

Afterword

1. Ruth W. Lidz, M.D., "Emotional Factors in the Success of Contraception," *Fertility and Sterility* 20, no. 5 (Sept.–Oct., 1969): 761. Also see "Conflicts Between Fertility and Infertility," to be published in *The Woman as a Patient*, C. Nadelson and M. Notman, eds., Plenum Publishing Co.

2. David A. Rodgers and Frederick J. Ziegler, "Psychological Reactions to Surgical Contraception," *Psychological Perspectives on Population*, James T. Fawcett, ed. (New York: Basic Books, 1973), pp. 306–325.

Index

abortions
  death rate from, 21
  septic, 18
abstinence
  for increased sperm count, 222,
    228
  learning to cope with, 72–5, 232
  marital disequilibrium caused
    by, 75–9
  marriages strengthened by, 4–5,
    63, 71, 74–5, 80–93, 103, 106,
    110–11, 191–3
  mutual responsibility for, 82–3,
    91–3, 97, 101–3, 108, 111
  post-Pill, 191–3
  sexual disequilibrium caused by,
    83–5
  and sexual dysfunction, 85–7
  and sexual energy control, 107–8,
    109
  studies on, 63–5
Anderman, Dr. Lester B., 229–30
anovulatory cycle, 193–6, 202
Applebaum, Dr. Richard M., 220–1

Bakker, Dr. Cornelius B., 98, 99
Bardwick, Dr. Judith M., 80, 98
Barglow, Dr. Peter, 66, 99, 100
Baylor College of Medicine, 26
Beral, Valerie, 15n, 28
Billings, Drs. John and Evelyn, 47
Brazelton, Dr. T. Berry, 207–8

breast-feeding, 207–21
  advantages, 207–13
  breast infection, 220–1
  convenience, 213–14
  frequency, 216
  full, 197, 200, 210, 216
  learning about, 214–21
  long-term effects, 212–13
  milk expression, 219–20
  and natural child-spacing, 62,
    197, 207–10, 216
  as ovulation suppressant, 198,
    199–201, 207–8, 210
  prolonged, 214
  sore nipples, 217–19
  weaning, 221
British Medical Journal, 15n, 25, 26
Busam, Dr. Paul A., 212
Byrne, Dr. Donn, 89

calendar rhythm, 65, 231–2
cervical changes
  charting, 180–5
  as fertility indicator, 53–7, 144–5,
    177–85, 188, 193, 194–6, 198, 201,
    204, 225
  hormonal effects on, 54–5
  and mucus changes, 55–6, 179–80
  during pre-menopause, 204
  post-partum, 198, 201
  recognizing, 56, 178–9
cervical mucus barrier, 36–7

248

254   *Index*

U.S. *Catholic*, 105
uterus, 33–4, 210

vagina, 34
vaginal
    deodorants, 124
    dryness, and infertility, 48
    secretions, 36
    See also cervical mucus
varicocele, 229
vasectomy, 24–7
    complications, 23, 25–6
    effectiveness of, 26–7
    procedure, 25–6
    reversal, 26–7
    shock factors in, 28, 70
    studies on, 25–6

Washington Post, 17
women
    equality for, and NFP, 5, 82–3,
        91–3
    fertility of, 34–6, 39–40, 117, 229–
        30, 233–4
    procreative function of, 223–4
    reproductive organs, 33–7, 117
    response to contraception, 7, 99,
        233
    responsibility for contraception,
        7, 10, 12–24, 66, 68, 70, 77–8,
        91–2, 97–9
    sexuality of, and abstinence, 81–
        93
    sterilization of, 19–24, 28, 223
    See also marriage; Ovulatory
        Phase; sexual relations